DIGITAL DATA IMPROVEMENT PRIORITIES FOR CONTINUOUS LEARNING IN HEALTH AND HEALTH CARE

Workshop Summary

Claudia Grossmann, Brian Powers, and Julia Sanders, *Rapporteurs*

Roundtable on Value & Science-Driven Health Care

INSTITUTE OF MEDICINE
OF THE NATIONAL ACADEMIES

THE NATIONAL ACADEMIES PRESS
Washington, D.C.
www.nap.edu

THE NATIONAL ACADEMIES PRESS   500 Fifth Street, NW   Washington, DC 20001

NOTICE: The project that is the subject of this report was approved by the Governing Board of the National Research Council, whose members are drawn from the councils of the National Academy of Sciences, the National Academy of Engineering, and the Institute of Medicine. The members of the committee responsible for the report were chosen for their special competences and with regard for appropriate balance.

This study was supported by Contract/Grant No. HHSP23320110009EC between the National Academy of Sciences and the Office of the National Coordinator for Health Information Technology. The views presented in this publication do not necessarily reflect the views of the organizations or agencies that provided support for the project.

International Standard Book Number-13:   978-0-309-25941-5
International Standard Book Number-10:   0-309-25941-X

Additional copies of this report are available for sale from the National Academies Press, 500 Fifth Street, NW, Keck 360, Washington, DC 20001; (800) 624-6242 or (202) 334-3313; http://www.nap.edu.

Copyright 2013 by the National Academy of Sciences. All rights reserved.

Printed in the United States of America

The serpent has been a symbol of long life, healing, and knowledge among almost all cultures and religions since the beginning of recorded history. The serpent adopted as a logotype by the Institute of Medicine is a relief carving from ancient Greece, now held by the Staatliche Museen in Berlin.

Suggested citation: IOM (Institute of Medicine). 2013. *Digital data improvement priorities for continuous learning in health and health care: Workshop summary.* Washington, DC: The National Academies Press.

"*Knowing is not enough; we must apply. Willing is not enough; we must do.*"
—Goethe

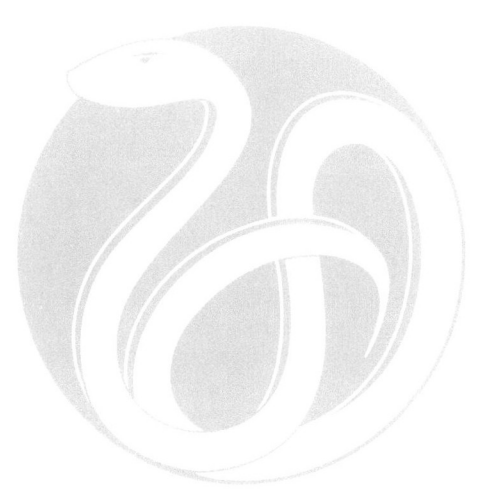

INSTITUTE OF MEDICINE
OF THE NATIONAL ACADEMIES

Advising the Nation. Improving Health.

THE NATIONAL ACADEMIES
Advisers to the Nation on Science, Engineering, and Medicine

The **National Academy of Sciences** is a private, nonprofit, self-perpetuating society of distinguished scholars engaged in scientific and engineering research, dedicated to the furtherance of science and technology and to their use for the general welfare. Upon the authority of the charter granted to it by the Congress in 1863, the Academy has a mandate that requires it to advise the federal government on scientific and technical matters. Dr. Ralph J. Cicerone is president of the National Academy of Sciences.

The **National Academy of Engineering** was established in 1964, under the charter of the National Academy of Sciences, as a parallel organization of outstanding engineers. It is autonomous in its administration and in the selection of its members, sharing with the National Academy of Sciences the responsibility for advising the federal government. The National Academy of Engineering also sponsors engineering programs aimed at meeting national needs, encourages education and research, and recognizes the superior achievements of engineers. Dr. Charles M. Vest is president of the National Academy of Engineering.

The **Institute of Medicine** was established in 1970 by the National Academy of Sciences to secure the services of eminent members of appropriate professions in the examination of policy matters pertaining to the health of the public. The Institute acts under the responsibility given to the National Academy of Sciences by its congressional charter to be an adviser to the federal government and, upon its own initiative, to identify issues of medical care, research, and education. Dr. Harvey V. Fineberg is president of the Institute of Medicine.

The **National Research Council** was organized by the National Academy of Sciences in 1916 to associate the broad community of science and technology with the Academy's purposes of furthering knowledge and advising the federal government. Functioning in accordance with general policies determined by the Academy, the Council has become the principal operating agency of both the National Academy of Sciences and the National Academy of Engineering in providing services to the government, the public, and the scientific and engineering communities. The Council is administered jointly by both Academies and the Institute of Medicine. Dr. Ralph J. Cicerone and Dr. Charles M. Vest are chair and vice chair, respectively, of the National Research Council.

www.national-academies.org

PLANNING COMMITTEE ON DIGITAL DATA PRIORITIES FOR CONTINUOUS LEARING[1]

JAMES WALKER (*Chair*), Chief Health Information Officer, Geisinger Health System
JUSTINE CARR, Chief Medical Officer, Steward Health Care
WILLIAM DuMOUCHEL, Chief Statistical Scientist, Oracle Health Sciences
JAMIE HEYWOOD, Chairman, PatientsLikeMe
REBECCA KUSH, President and CEO, Clinical Data Standards Interchange Consortium
LISA LEE, Chief Science Officer, Office of Surveillance, Epidemiology, and Laboratory Sciences, Centers for Disease Control and Prevention
THERESA MULLIN, Director, Office of Planning and Informatics, Center for Drug Evaluation and Research, Food and Drug Administration
LUCILA OHNO-MACHADO, Founding Chief, Biomedical Informatics, University of California, San Diego
RICHARD PLATT, Chair, Population Medicine, Harvard University
JIM SCANLON, Deputy Assistant Secretary for Planning and Evaluation (Science and Policy), U.S. Department of Health and Human Services
PAUL STANG, Senior Director of Epidemeology, Johnson & Johnson
WALTER SUAREZ, Director, Health IT Strategy and Policy, Kaiser Permanente

IOM Staff

CLAUDIA GROSSMANN, Senior Program Officer
BRIAN POWERS, Senior Program Assistant (through July 2012)
VALERIE ROHRBACH, Senior Program Assistant
JULIA SANDERS, Senior Program Assistant
ROBERT SAUNDERS, Study Director
LEIGH STUCKHARDT, Program Associate
ISABELLE VON KOHORN, Program Officer
BARRET ZIMMERMANN, Program Assistant
J. MICHAEL McGINNIS, Senior Scholar, Executive Director, Roundtable on Value & Science-Driven Health Care

---

[1] Institute of Medicine planning committees are solely responsible for organizing the workshop, identifying topics, and choosing speakers. The responsibility for the published workshop summary rests with the workshop rapporteurs and the institution.

ROUNDTABLE ON VALUE & SCIENCE-DRIVEN HEALTH CARE[1]

MARK B. McCLELLAN (*Chair*), Director, Engelberg Center, The Brookings Institution
DAVID BLUMENTHAL, President, The Commonwealth Fund
BRUCE G. BODAKEN, Chairman, President, and CEO, Blue Shield of California
PAUL CHEW, Chief Science Officer and Chief Medical Officer, Sanofi U.S.
CAROLYN M. CLANCY, Director, Agency for Healthcare Research and Quality (Ex Officio)
FRANCIS COLLINS, Director, National Institutes of Health (Ex Officio) (*designee:* **Susan Shurin**)
HELEN DARLING, President, National Business Group on Health
SUSAN D. DEVORE, Chief Executive Officer, Premier, Inc.
RICHARD FANTE, Regional VP, Americans, AstraZeneca
JUDITH FAULKNER, Founder and CEO, Epic Health Systems
THOMAS R. FRIEDEN, Director, Centers for Disease Control and Prevention (Ex Officio) (*designee:* **Gail R. Janes**)
PATRICIA A. GABOW, CEO, Denver Health
ATUL GAWANDE, General and Endocrine Surgeon, Brigham and Women's Hospital
GARY L. GOTTLIEB, President and CEO, Partners HealthCare System
JAMES A. GUEST, President, Consumers Union
GEORGE C. HALVORSON, Chairman and CEO, Kaiser Permanente
MARGARET A. HAMBURG, Commissioner, Food and Drug Administration (Ex Officio) (*designee:* **Peter Lurie**)
JAMES HEYWOOD, Co-Founder and Chairman, PatientsLikeMe
RALPH I. HORWITZ, Senior VP, Clinical Evaluation Sciences, GlaxoSmithKline
BRENT C. JAMES, Chief Quality Officer and Executive Director, Institute for Health Care Delivery Research, Intermountain Healthcare
MICHAEL M. E. JOHNS, Chancellor, Emory University
CRAIG JONES, Director, Vermont Blueprint for Health
GARY KAPLAN, Chairman and CEO, Virginia Mason Health System
RICHARD C. LARSON, Mitsui Professor, Massachusetts Institute of Technology
JAMES L. MADARA, CEO, American Medical Association

---

[1] Institute of Medicine forums and roundtables do not issue, review, or approve individual documents. The responsibility for the published workshop summary rests with the workshop rapporteurs and the institution.

FARZAD MOSTASHARI, National Coordinator, Office of the National Coordinator for Health IT (Ex Officio)
MARY D. NAYLOR, Professor and Director, Center for Transitions in Health, University of Pennsylvania
WILLIAM D. NOVELLI, Former CEO, AARP; Professor, Georgetown University
SAM NUSSBAUM, Executive VP, Clinical Health Policy and Chief Medical Officer, WellPoint, Inc.
JONATHAN B. PERLIN, Chief Medical Officer and President, Clinical & Physician Services, Hospital Corporation of America, Inc.
ROBERT A. PETZEL, Under Secretary for Health, Department of Veterans Affairs (Ex Officio)
RICHARD PLATT, Professor and Chair, Population Medicine, Harvard Medical School
JOHN W. ROWE, Professor, Mailman School of Public Health, Columbia University
JOE SELBY, Executive Director, PCORI
MARK D. SMITH, President and CEO, California HealthCare Foundation
GLENN D. STEELE, President and CEO, Geisinger Health System
MARILYN TAVENNER, Administrator, Centers for Medicare & Medicaid Services (Ex Officio) (*designee:* **Patrick Conway**)
REED D. TUCKSON, Executive VP and Chief of Medical Affairs, UnitedHealth Group
MARY WAKEFIELD, Administrator, Health Resources and Services Administration (Ex Officio)
DEBRA B. WHITMAN, Executive Vice President, Policy and International, AARP
JONATHAN WOODSON, Assistant Secretary for Health, Department of Defense (Ex Officio)

Institute of Medicine
Roundtable on Value & Science-Driven Health Care
Charter and Vision Statement

The Institute of Medicine's Roundtable on Value & Science-Driven Health Care has been convened to help transform the way evidence on clinical effectiveness is generated and used to improve health and health care. Participants have set a goal that, by the year 2020, 90 percent of clinical decisions will be supported by accurate, timely, and up-to-date clinical information, and will reflect the best available evidence. Roundtable members will work with their colleagues to identify the issues not being adequately addressed, the nature of the barriers and possible solutions, and the priorities for action, and will marshal the resources of the sectors represented on the Roundtable to work for sustained public–private cooperation for change.

****

Vision: Our vision is for the development of a continuously learning health system in which science, informatics, incentives, and culture are aligned for continuous improvement and innovation—with best practices seamlessly embedded in the care process and new knowledge captured as an integral by-product of the care experience.

Goal: By the year 2020, 90 percent of clinical decisions will be supported by accurate, timely, and up-to-date clinical information, and will reflect the best available evidence. We feel that this presents a tangible focus for progress toward our vision, that Americans ought to expect at least this level of performance, that it should be feasible with existing resources and emerging tools, and that measures can be developed to track and stimulate progress.

Context: As unprecedented developments in the diagnosis, treatment, and long-term management of disease bring Americans closer than ever to the promise of personalized health care, we are faced with similarly unprecedented challenges to identify and deliver the care most appropriate for individual needs and conditions. Care that is important is often not delivered. Care that is delivered is often not important. In part, this is due to our failure to apply the evidence we have about the medical care that is most effective—a failure related to shortfalls in provider knowledge and accountability, inadequate care coordination and support, lack of insurance, poorly aligned payment incentives, and misplaced patient expectations. Increasingly, it is also a result of our limited capacity for timely generation of evidence on the relative effectiveness, efficiency, and safety of available and emerging interventions. Improving the value of the return on our healthcare investment is a vital imperative that will require much greater capacity to evaluate high priority clinical interventions, stronger links between clinical research and practice, and reorientation of the incentives to apply new insights. We must quicken our efforts to position evidence development and application as natural outgrowths of clinical care—to foster health care that learns.

Approach: The IOM Roundtable on Value & Science-Driven Health Care serves as a forum to facilitate the collaborative assessment and action around issues central to achieving the vision and goal stated. The challenges are myriad and include issues that must be addressed to improve evidence development, evidence application, and the capacity to advance progress on both dimensions. To address these challenges, as leaders in their fields, Roundtable members work with their colleagues to identify the issues not being adequately addressed, the nature of the barriers and possible solutions, and the priorities for action, and marshal the resources of the sectors represented on the Roundtable to work for sustained public-private cooperation for change. Activities include collaborative exploration of new and expedited approaches to assessing the effectiveness of diagnostic and treatment interventions, better use of the patient care experience to generate evidence on effectiveness and efficiency of care, identification of assessment priorities, and communication strategies to enhance provider and patient understanding and support for interventions proven to work best and deliver value in health care.

Core concepts and principles: For the purpose of the Roundtable activities, we define science-driven health care broadly to mean that, to the greatest extent possible, the decisions that shape the health and health care of Americans—by patients, providers, payers and policymakers alike—will be grounded on a reliable evidence base, will account appropriately for individual variation in patient needs, and will support the generation of new insights on clinical effectiveness. Evidence is generally considered to be information from clinical experience that has met some established test of validity, and the appropriate standard is determined according to the requirements of the intervention and clinical circumstance. Processes that involve the development and use of evidence should be accessible and transparent to all stakeholders.

A common commitment to certain principles and priorities guides the activities of the Roundtable and its members, including the commitment to: the right health care for each person; putting the best evidence into practice; establishing the effectiveness, efficiency and safety of medical care delivered; building constant measurement into our healthcare investments; the establishment of healthcare data as a public good; shared responsibility distributed equitably across stakeholders, both public and private; collaborative stakeholder involvement in priority setting; transparency in the execution of activities and reporting of results; and subjugation of individual political or stakeholder perspectives in favor of the common good.

Reviewers

This workshop summary has been reviewed in draft form by individuals chosen for their diverse perspectives and technical expertise, in accordance with procedures approved by the National Research Council's Report Review Committee. The purpose of this independent review is to provide candid and critical comments that will assist the institution in making its published workshop summary as sound as possible and to ensure that the workshop summary meets institutional standards for objectivity, evidence, and responsiveness to the study charge. The review comments and draft manuscript remain confidential to protect the integrity of the process. We wish to thank the following individuals for their review of this workshop summary:

Alfred DeMaria, Massachusetts Department of Public Health
Shaun Grannis, Regenstrief Institute, Inc.
Erin Holve, AcademyHealth
Jonathan Silverstein, NorthShore University Health System

Although the reviewers listed above have provided many constructive comments and suggestions, they did not see the final draft of the workshop summary before its release. The review of this workshop summary was overseen by **Joy Keeler Tobin,** MITRE. Appointed by the Institute of Medicine, she was responsible for making certain that an independent examination of this workshop summary was carried out in accordance with institutional procedures and that all review comments were carefully considered. Responsibility for the final content of this workshop summary rests entirely with the authors and the institution.

Preface

In light of the challenges and opportunities associated with the increasing amount of digital health and health-related information being generated and collected in modern society, the Institute of Medicine's Roundtable on Value & Science-Driven Health Care, with the support of the Office of the National Coordinator for Health Information Technology, convened a workshop on Digital Data Priorities for Continuous Learning in Health and Health Care, which is summarized in this publication. Experts from a wide range of disciplines—including medicine, public health, informatics, health information technology, health care services research, health care quality reporting, biomedical research, clinical research, statistics, medical product manufacturing, health care payment and financing, and patient advocacy—met to explore the data quality issues and strategies central to the increasing capture and use of digital health data for knowledge development. This publication summarizes discussions to clarify understanding of, and accelerate progress around, data improvement priorities for the digital health data utility.

The vision of the Roundtable is for a health system in which learning is continuous, with medical evidence generated by capturing the care experience and applied to ensure and improve best care practices. Since its inception in 2006, the Roundtable has set out to help realize this vision through the involvement and support of senior leadership from key health care stakeholders. In engaging the nation's leaders in workshops and other activities, Roundtable members and colleagues provide guidance on issues important to advancing the development and use of a digital health data utility for knowledge generation and continuous improvement.

Building on this groundwork, the objectives of this workshop were to identify and characterize the current deficiencies in the reliability, availability, and usability of digital health data and consider strategies, priorities, and responsibilities to address such deficiencies. Content was structured to explore the data quality challenges and opportunities in a learning health system associated with population and care process management, clinical research, translational informatics, and public health support at the national and state level. Workshop discussion also explored the potential for learning from large-scale health datasets, focusing on innovative approaches to overcoming the challenges of distributed data, data harmonization, and identity resolution.

Multiple individuals donated valuable time toward the development of this publication. *We would like to acknowledge and offer strong appreciation for the contributors to this volume for their presence at the workshop and their efforts to further develop their presentations into the summaries contained in this publication.* We are especially indebted to those who provided counsel by serving on the planning committee for this workshop, including Justine Carr (Steward Health Care), William DuMouchel (Oracle Health Sciences), Jamie Heywood (PatientsLikeMe), Rebecca Kush (Clinical Data Standards Interchange Consortium), Lisa Lee (CDC, Office of Surveillance, Epidemiology, and Laboratory Services), Theresa Mullin (FDA, Center for Drug Evaluation and Research), Lucila Ohno-Machado (University of California, San Diego), Richard Platt (Harvard University), Jim Scanlon (Department of Health and Human Services), Paul Stang (Johnson & Johnson), and Walter Suarez (Kaiser Permanente).

Under the leadership of senior program officer Claudia Grossmann, a number of Roundtable staff played instrumental roles in coordinating the workshop and translating the workshop proceedings into this summary, including Brian Powers, Valerie Rohrbach, Julia Sanders, Robert Saunders, Leigh Stuckhardt, and Isabelle Von Kohorn. We would also like to thank Daniel Bethea, Laura Harbold DeStefano, Christine Stencel, and Sarah Ziegenhorn for helping to coordinate various aspects of review, production, and publication.

Reliable digital health data represent the foundational elements of a continuously learning health system. The discussions summarized in this workshop explore the potential and challenges for utilizing these data for learning and outline potential strategies and actions to catalyze progress.

We believe *Digital Data Improvement Priorities for Continuous Learning in Health and Health Care* will be a valuable resource as efforts to build and leverage the digital health data utility continue to move forward.

James Walker, *Chair*
Planning Committee on
Digital Data Priorities for Continuous Learning
Chief Health Information Officer
Geisinger Health System

J. Michael McGinnis
Senior Scholar
Executive Director
Roundtable on Value & Science-Driven Health Care
Institute of Medicine

Contents

1 **Introduction**   1
Data Sources in the Digital Health Utility, 3
Moving to a Continuously Learning Health System, 4
Workshop Scope and Objectives, 5
Organization of the Summary, 6

2 **Data Quality Challenges and Opportunities in a Learning Health System**   9
Introduction, 10
Challenges for Data Collection and Aggregation, 10
Patient-Reported Data and Maximizing Patient Value in the Learning Health System, 12

3 **Digital Health Data Uses: Leveraging Data for Better Health**   15
Introduction, 17
Practice Management, 17
Clinical Research, 19
Translational Informatics, 21
Supporting Public Health and Surveillance at the National Level, 23
Supporting Public Health and Surveillance at the Local Level, 24

4	**Issues and Opportunities in the Emergence of Large Health-Related Datasets** Introduction, 28 The Challenge of Bias in Large Health-Related Datasets, 28 Moving from Analytics to Insights, 30	27
5	**Innovations Emerging in the Clinical Data Utility** Introduction, 34 Distributed Queries, 34 Data Harmonization and Normalization, 36 Data Linkage, 38	33
6	**Strategies Going Forward** Current Data Sources: Better Awareness and Assessment, 41 Data Input: Improve Patient Orientation, Quality, and Utility, 42 Data Analysis: Improve Access, Tools, and Capacity, 42 Public and Patient Engagement: Ramp Up Involvement, 43 Building a Clinical Data Learning Utility, 44 Clarity on Governance, 45	41

Appendixes

A	Speaker Biographies	47
B	Workshop Agenda	57

1

Introduction

Digital health data are the lifeblood of a continuous learning health system. A steady flow of reliable data is necessary to coordinate and monitor patient care, analyze and improve systems of care, conduct research to develop new products and approaches, assess the effectiveness of medical interventions, and advance population health. The totality of available health data is a crucial resource that should be considered an invaluable public asset in the pursuit of better care, improved health, and lower health care costs (IOM, 2012). This publication summarizes discussions at the March 2012 Institute of Medicine (IOM) workshop to identify and characterize the current deficiencies in the reliability, availability, and usability of digital health data and consider strategies, priorities, and responsibilities to address such deficiencies.[1]

The ability to collect, share, and use digital health data is rapidly evolving. Increasing adoption of electronic health records (EHRs) is being driven by the implementation of the Health Information Technology for Economic and Clinical Health (HITECH) Act, which pays hospitals and individuals incentives if they can demonstrate that they use EHRs in a meaningful way. However, although more than half of office-based physicians were using basic EHRs in 2011, only a third had access to the basic features necessary

---

[1] The planning committee's role was limited to planning the workshop, and the workshop summary has been prepared by the workshop rapporteurs as a factual summary of what occurred at the workshop. Statements, recommendations, and opinions expressed are those of individual presenters and participants, and are not necessarily endorsed or verified by the Institute of Medicine, and they should not be construed as reflecting any group consensus.

to leverage this information for improvement, such as the ability to view laboratory results, maintain problem lists, or manage prescription ordering, (Decker et al., 2012).

In addition to increased data collection, more organizations are sharing digital health data. Data collected to meet federal reporting requirements or for administrative purposes are becoming more accessible. Efforts such as Health.Data.gov provide access to government datasets for the development of insights and software applications with the goal of improving health. Within the private sector, at least one pharmaceutical company is actively exploring release of some of its clinical trial data for research by others.[2] Data sharing partnerships are also opening up across organizations. The Care Connectivity Consortium, a group of five health systems at the leading edge of using EHRs (Kaiser Permanente, Geisinger Health System, Mayo Clinic, Intermoutain Healthcare, and Group Health Cooperative), have agreed to securely exchange clinical data for care coordination. Sharing is also happening across industries. In the case of AstraZeneca and WellPoint, a payer and a product manufacturer have initiated a study on the clinical and cost effectiveness of treatments for some chronic and common diseases. Finally, efforts to increase patient access to their own data, such as the Blue Button initiative which allows patients to download their health information with the click of a button, have been adopted by organizations such as the Veterans Health Administration and UnitedHealthcare, and included in the criteria for Meaningful Use.

The increased collection and sharing of health data is quickly moving health care into the era of "big data." This term refers to the huge volume and diversity of data collected in increasingly connected digital technologies. The scale of "big data" has implications for analysis and learning in a way that has been leveraged by other industries, such as intelligence, but is only beginning in health care.

Increasing collection, sharing, and aggregation of data are being matched by advances in methods for learning from these data. Clinical and administrative data can be used for studies to assess the effectiveness of health care interventions; identify product safety issues; detect emerging epidemics; and measure health care utilization and value. Observational methods that use data collected in the course of providing patient care are increasingly appreciated as valuable contributors to generating and testing hypotheses. The rapidly rising costs and extended duration of traditional randomized control trials (RCTs) have contributed to the interests of investigators and funders, among whom there is a growing appreciation of the need to harness big data for innovative streamlined approaches to testing new interventions.

---

[2] Personal communication, Joel Beetsch, Sanofi.

Crucial to all of these efforts is the appropriate alignment of data sources with their intended use. Different uses have different requirements of data, and therefore different priorities in terms of the evolving clinical data utility. This challenge is magnified by the lack of lessons and best practices for how to approach data quality assurances needed to support the multiple facets of a learning health system. To address these issues and gain a better understanding of the types, sources, applications, limitations, appropriate uses, and quality improvement needs for digital health data, the IOM's Roundtable on Value & Science-Driven Health Care convened a meeting on March 23, 2012, titled Digital Data Priorities for Continuous Learning in Health and Health Care. This meeting followed a series of related discussions summarized in the IOM publication titled *Digital Infrastructure for the Learning Health System* (2011), and built on a body of work done by the Roundtable on the centrality of a clinical data utility to support continuous learning and improvement in health and health care (IOM, 2010, 2011a,b,c).

DATA SOURCES IN THE DIGITAL HEALTH UTILITY

Digital health data are produced in a variety of different environments, which impact greatly the characteristics of the data. Who collects the data, how it is collected, why it is collected, and what is collected are some of the ways that digital health data differ depending on their source and have implications for the use of that data. Understanding these characteristics is necessary to match data users with appropriate sources, and to understand limitations and barriers in data analysis.

The increased adoption of EHRs has given data from routine care increasing prominence as a potential component of the data utility. Data collected in the course of delivering patient care come from a variety of sources such as clinician offices, ambulatory procedure centers, hospitals, and nursing and extended care facilities. The types of data vary by care setting, but generally include both clinical and administrative elements. Clinical elements include structured fields and free text notes, laboratory results, images, and diagnostic test results. Administrative information includes process performance metrics, and details needed for billing, such as International Classification of Diseases (ICD) codes.

Also growing in importance is data originating directly from patients. These data can be captured through the use of personal health records or patient portals, in clinical records as recorded by healthcare personnel, or in records external to the health system. They can include personal reports of current health status and wellness, family history, and remote site laboratory readings, as well as health-related data such as socioeconomic, environmental, and lifestyle factors. There is increasing interest in including patient-generated data in data sources such as the use of patient-reported outcomes in research studies.

Ongoing and completed clinical trial data offer yet another major source of new data insights—even beyond the immediate study focus. Trials funded by public or private sponsors are largely carried out either at academic institutions or in community settings. Clinical trial data are typically collected in addition to those already collected in routine care, usually follow a standardized protocol, and are recorded in a case report form. When the trial is performed for the approval or assessment of a regulated medical product such as a new drug or device, the Food and Drug Administration (FDA) closely regulates how and what data are collected. In addition to traditional clinical trials, registries for quality activities, research, or post-marketing surveillance are a parallel source of enriched clinical data.

Employers, as the purchasers of health insurance for much of the population, often possess data on employees' health care utilization, basic health status, and associated expenses which can be used for knowledge development. In addition, these data can have greater longitudinal richness than records from clinical care providers.

A final source of health data is population health data routinely collected through the public health system and its surveys and surveillance activities. These data provide information on overall health trends, such as births and deaths, disease prevalence, community health, environmental health, and access to care, as well as disease incidence and threat data. The collection and reporting of this information is increasingly digital, either through freestanding systems and portals or as integrated parts of EHR systems. Given the many levels at which public health works—local, county, state, and federal—different data collection approaches and requirements exist at the different levels. Other health-related community level data are routinely collected by various organizations, departments, and agencies. This includes community socioeconomic status profile data; community physical profile data, such as density, design, and use; civic engagement profiles; and community employer profile. Additionally, organizations collect data on individuals through their commercial and social activities, such as through supermarket rewards programs and Web-surfing patterns. These data are used not only on their own, for insights into the community, but in concert with other health data to yield a more complete understanding of population health.

MOVING TO A CONTINUOUSLY LEARNING HEALTH SYSTEM

Although the collection of large amounts of health and health-related data holds promise for both the scale and types of learning possible, data alone are not sufficient for learning. Sharing, aggregation, analysis, and the continuous management and improvement of these data are necessary to enable the transition to a continuously learning health system.

The applications of digital health data in a learning system are multiple, including care coordination; management of patient populations; associated care and business processes; outcome, quality, and value assessments; generation of clinical evidence, including clinical trials, clinical effectiveness, and genomic studies; surveillance and trend detection, including medical products safety, syndromic and actionable surveillance, and hypothesis generation; and public health program management. These differing uses vary in their requirements for data quality and characteristics, but all share common challenges related to data access, liquidity, interoperability, and the development of innovative methods for analysis. These issues formed the foundation for the presentations and discussions at the IOM public workshop on Digital Data Priorities for Continuous Learning in Health and Health Care.

WORKSHOP SCOPE AND OBJECTIVES

Workshop participants included experts from across medicine, public health, informatics, health information technology, health care services research, health care quality reporting, biomedical research, clinical research, statistics, medical product manufacturing, health care payment and financing, and patient advocacy. Content was structured to explore the data quality challenges and opportunities in a learning health system, highlighting the opportunities and priorities beyond care coordination such as population and care process management, clinical research, translational informatics, and public health support at the national and state level. The workshop also explored the potential for learning from large-scale health datasets, focusing on innovative approaches to overcoming the challenges of distributed data, data harmonization, and identity resolution.

The workshop statement of task can be found in Box 1-1, and the elements are reflected in the stated meeting objectives:

1. Discuss the current quality status of digital health data.
2. Explore challenges, and identify key questions related to data quality in the use of EHRs, patient registries, administrative data, and public health sources for learning—continuous and episodic—and for system operational and improvement purposes.
3. Engage individuals and organizations leading the way in improving the reliability, availability, and usability of digital health data for real-time knowledge generation and health improvement in a continuously learning health system.

> **BOX 1-1**
> **Statement of Task**
>
> An ad hoc committee will plan and conduct a public workshop to explore the data quality issues and strategies central to the increasing capture and use of digital clinical and patient-reported data for knowledge development. The workshop will engage leading experts in reviewing the challenges, defining key questions, and exploring a strategic framework for progress on the issue of health data quality in a learning health system. Questions/topics of consideration could include What are the data quality requirements to support the various knowledge generation processes required by the learning health system (quality monitoring, sentinel event detection, disease surveillance, clinical research)? What is known about the current state of digital health data quality? What implications does this have for short term uses? What analytical methods are available to assess data quality? What novel analytical methods will need to be developed in order to meet learning health system data-use needs? What are the essential components of a strategy to achieve the necessary data quality levels? What lessons have been learned by those organizations already undertaking learning health system–type efforts? What foundational work has been done that can be built on/leveraged to better meet learning health system data quality needs?

4. Identify and characterize the current deficiencies and consider strategies, priorities, and responsibilities to address the deficiencies.
5. Initiate the development of a strategic framework for integrated and networked stewardship of efforts to continuously increase digital data utility.

Through a series of expert presentations and discussions, workshop participants addressed issues of matching data quality to use, how these needs align with current data sources, and what the potential and challenges are for leveraging digital health data for learning—both the short and long term. The final workshop session included a moderated discussion geared toward describing ways forward on the issues highlighted earlier in the workshop.

ORGANIZATION OF THE SUMMARY

This publication summarizes the proceedings of the workshop on Digital Data Priorities for Continuous Learning in Health and Health Care, the 12th in the Learning Health System Series of publications by the Roundtable on Value & Science-Driven Health Care. Chapters 2 through 5 summarize the expert presentations at the workshop, and are organized by thematic focus on the presentations, while Chapter 6 covers the concluding discussion. Chapter 2 addresses data quality challenges and opportunities in a learning health system, including explorations of data heterogeneity and the importance of focusing on data of value to the patient. Chapter 3 focuses on the many uses of the digital health data utility, covering the management of patient populations, clinical research, translational informatics, and both national and local public health efforts. Chapter 4 looks at emerging issues and opportunities in the use of large datasets, including a discussion of the challenge of data bias, and recent advances in mathematics that promise to move research toward generating real time insights. Chapter 5 explores emerging innovations in the use of digital health data including distributed queries, data normalization, and data linkages. Chapter 6 summarizes the concluding discussion in which many workshop participants suggested potential strategies and actions to catalyze progress.

REFERENCES

Decker, S. L., E. W. Jamoom, and J. E. Sisk. 2012. Physicians in nonprimary care and small practices and those age 55 and older lag in adopting electronic health record systems. *Health Affairs* 31(5):1-7.

IOM (Institute of Medicine). 2010. *Redesigning the clinical effectiveness research paradigm: Innovation and practice-based approaches.* Washington, DC: The National Academies Press.

———. 2011a. *Clinical data as the basic staple for health learning: Creating and protecting a public good.* Washington, DC: The National Academies Press.

———. 2011b. *Digital infrastructure for the learning health system: The road to continuous improvement in health and health care.* Washington, DC: The National Academies Press.

———. 2011c. *Learning what works: Infrastructure required for comparative effectiveness research.* Washington, DC: The National Academies Press.

2

Data Quality Challenges and Opportunities in a Learning Health System

---

KEY SPEAKER THEMES

Overhage

- Heterogeneity of data limits the ability to draw conclusions across datasets.
- Data quality assessment requires understanding if data is fit for its intended purpose.
- Data collection should aim to maximize value by balancing the burden of collection with its usefulness.

Heywood

- Clinical research is not currently focused on what patients consider valuable.
- Patient-reported data are critical for answering questions important to patients.
- A learning health system will require converging clinical research and clinical care on a common platform constantly oriented around patient value.

INTRODUCTION

A learning health system relies on collecting and aggregating a variety of clinical data sources at the patient, practice, and population level. Realizing this goal requires addressing concerns over data quality and harnessing new opportunities and sources of clinically relevant data. Marc Overhage, Chief Medical Informatics Officer at Siemens Healthcare, focused his presentation on the challenges for data collections and the limitations inherent in aggregating data across sources. Jamie Heywood, Co-Founder and Chairman of PatientsLikeMe, examined the issue of data quality as it relates to patient-reported data, and how patient value must be a central strategy in building a learning health system.

CHALLENGES FOR DATA COLLECTION AND AGGREGATION

Marc Overhage focused on several of the challenges posed by collecting and aggregating data to help derive meaningful conclusions and improve care. At each possible source of data collection, he noted, there are limitations to the quality of data obtained. With patient reported data, the way a patient understands or reports an event may not be understood in the same way by clinicians or researchers. Clinician-recorded data is limited in scope and quality by the time it takes to input structured data into an EHR. Finally, while external sources of data—labs, imaging, pharmacy, etc.—are not subject to the same human biases, they still carry other biases and limitations such as lack of standardization across products.

Overhage focused on structured data collection from the clinician perspective, which he posed as a balance between the burden and cost associated with its collection (impact on usability) and its value (usefulness of data) (see Figure 2-1). More structured data is generally more useful. However, the level of structure dramatically impacts the burden of collection, and therefore the usability of the collection system; rigidly structured data is usually time- and resource-intensive to collect. There should be a focus on maximizing both usability and usefulness—that is, finding optimum value.

Structured data collection is only part of the challenge. According to Overhage, although more and more efforts are being made to bring data together in a "queryable well," most digital health data remains siloed within different institutions and organizations. Data aggregation is crucial for a learning health system, but brings about new challenges.

One challenge noted by Overhage is the ability to identify patients across sources. When health information exchanges combine data from various sources, duplication of data or different views of the same clinical event can occur. He brought up the example of identifying which patients are on statins. Patients can be identified either based on medication order

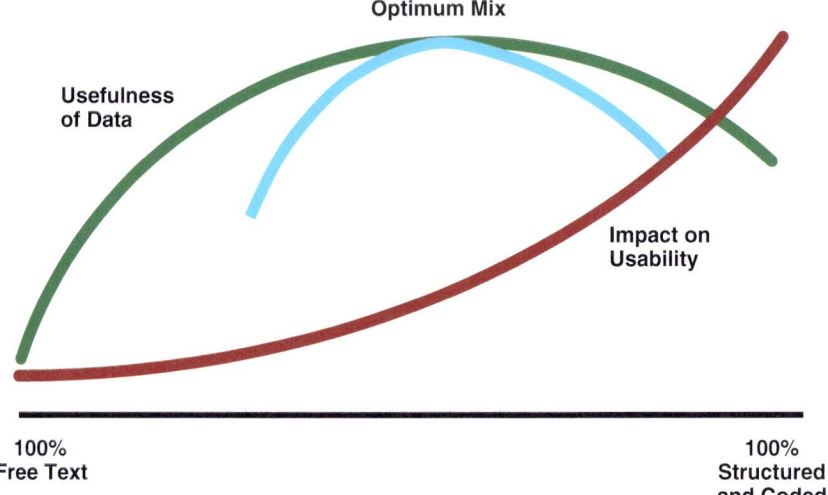

FIGURE 2-1 The usability-usefulness tradeoff for data collection.
SOURCE: From Ambulatory practice clinical information management: Problems and prospects, by B. Middleton, K. Renner, and M. Leavitt. *Journal of Healthcare Information Management* 11(4):97-112. Copyright 2012 by the Healthcare Information and Management Systems Society. Adapted with permission.

data from an EHR or by claims data. Both are "right," as both are facts about the patient, but they can yield different results. Some patients have both an ordering event and a dispensing event, some have one or the other, and some have neither. Successful data aggregation, according to Overhage, will need to account for the fact that there are going to be repeated observations and conflicting evidence, and combine evidence in a meaningful way. Fortunately, there are computational advances that can improve this process. Overhage pointed to work being done at Siemens on computer algorithms that can parse through conflicting evidence, assess its provenance, and begin to draw conclusions that clinicians can use.

Another challenge cited by Overhage was the ability to conduct population-level research on interventions and outcomes. He expressed caution with using large claims or health system EHR databases to draw conclusions. In particular, he focused on the importance of understanding the characteristics of datasets, such as the underrepresentation of females in the Department of Veterans Affairs (VA), especially when making comparisons across datasets. He presented data from the Observational Medical Outcomes Partnership (OMOP) showing the correlation of Cox-2 inhibitor use to an increased incidence of myocardial infarction in a health system dataset. When this correlation was explored in other health system and claims datasets, however, no relationship was found. This type of heterogeneity impacts efforts to combine datasets for observational research. Differences in context and demographics limit comparability between datasets. For example, Medicare has a vastly different age distribution than most commercial payers. Similarly, the gender distribution for the VA dataset is disproportionately skewed toward males. Heterogeneity is not limited to demographics, he stressed, but also includes the context in which the data was collected—e.g., changes in drug utilization patterns within a given health system over time.

Overhage concluded his remarks by stressing the need to appreciate that data quality lies in the eye of the beholder. The true quality of digital health data is an assessment of whether they are fit for their intended purpose. For example, he noted, data quality for population health measurement may be able to tolerate more error since researchers are looking for trends and changes at the population level. The same may be true for quality-measure adherence as well. However, at the individual patient encounter, decision support needs to be exactly right, and clinicians must have the correct information on the correct patient. Depending on the use, criteria for what is "good-enough" data will vary tremendously.

PATIENT-REPORTED DATA AND MAXIMIZING PATIENT VALUE IN THE LEARNING HEALTH SYSTEM

Heywood began his presentation with a series of quotes from management expert Peter Drucker: (1) Who is your customer? (2) What does your customer consider value? and (3) What are your results with customers? He proposed that the fact that health care costs have been increasing while the value of care has been decreasing can be traced to an inability to understand and answer these questions in the health care system.

In health care, Heywood stressed, the patient is the customer. This relationship, however, can be obscured in the research setting. According to Heywood, the clinician or researcher asking the question, rather than the patients, can often become the customer. This has profound implications on the utility of research. If the patient is the customer, he noted, research should be delivering results that they consider valuable. Currently, this is often not the case. Most clinical research focuses on physiologic, molecular, and other markers rather than aspects that matter most to patients: well-being and productivity. In order to serve their customers most effectively, Heywood proposed that all of research should be helping to answer this question that patients value most: *Given my status, what is the best outcome I could hope to achieve and how do I get there?* Digital health data that help to answer this question needs to be captured, recorded, and analyzed.

According to Heywood, patient-reported data can help improve the relevance of medical research to patients. He provided a brief overview of the PatientsLikeMe (PLM) online platform, and how it enables patients to share their data and learn from others. Patients create profiles on PLM which detail personal information, medical history, treatment history, and track functional status over time (using accepted patient reported outcome measures). This allows other patients on the site to find individuals similar to them, and learn from their experiences.

Despite some concerns over the perceived quality of patient reported data, Heywood provided an example of how patient-reported data can answer some of the same questions that traditional clinical outcomes research methods are used for. Since patients with amyotrophic lateral sclerosis (ALS) comprise one of the largest groups on PLM, he detailed the use of patient-reported data to assess the efficacy of lithium in slowing the progression of ALS. In 2008, the results of a clinical trial were published showing that lithium significantly slowed the progression of ALS symptoms. Using the PLM platform, researchers were able to test this same treatment in the PLM population. They used an algorithm to match ALS patients being treated with lithium to similar patients who were not undergoing lithium treatment. The variety of demographic and physiologic variables recorded on PLM profiles allowed for each patient to be matched to an individual control, rather than pairing groups. No change in the progression of ALS symptoms was observed in the population being treated with lithium. The same results were later found in four clinical trials stopped early for futility.

The benefit of routinely collecting patient-reported data through a platform like PLM is that it greatly speeds up the assessment process for interventions. Since data are already in place, conducting clinical research does not require building new infrastructure nor collecting new data. According to Heywood, this allowed the researchers at PLM to conduct their study of lithium efficacy in ALS patients in a fraction of the time, and at a fraction of the cost, of the follow-up clinical trials to the 2008 study.

After focusing on the ALS case study, Heywood broadened his discussion to consider the transformation necessary to use data—regardless of source—to improve the health system. He returned to the center question patients value most: Given my status, what is the best outcome I could hope to achieve and how do I get there? The path to answering this question, he suggested, is building learning mechanisms, such as predictive models, into the system to speed discovery, assessment, and implementation. If done effectively, this would converge clinical research and clinical care into one model on a common platform. Heywood proposed that if this is done within the context of what the patient perceives as valuable, and keeps

14 DIGITAL DATA IMPROVEMENT PRIORITIES

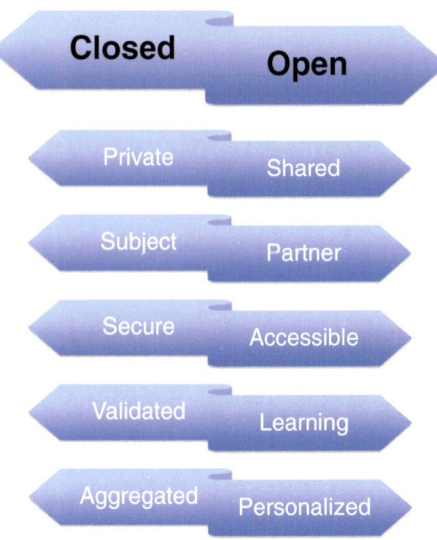

FIGURE 2-2 Paradigm shifts required for the realization of a learning health system. Status quo is presented on the left and requirements of a learning health system on the right.
SOURCE: Reprinted with permission from James Heywood.

patients part of the process the whole time, the result will be a learning health system. Heywood concluded his remarks with a series of paradigm shifts necessary to move toward a learning health system (Figure 2-2). These include moving toward a system characterized by sharing rather than privatization, patients as partners rather than subjects in research, accessibility rather than security, learning rather than validation, personalization rather than aggregation, and openness rather than closedness.

3

Digital Health Data Uses: Leveraging Data for Better Health

KEY SPEAKER THEMES

Leenay

- Shared information in health care must evolve to include all stakeholders as active constituents in the health care conversation.
- Data included in current digital record systems must be more accurate, timely, and standardized to support actionable decisions.
- ACOs represent an alignment of incentives for the collection of higher-quality data, with greater completeness and accuracy, and the increased liquidity of this data.

Kush

- Data standards are key to improving data quality.
- Quality must be built into research methods from the beginning.
- Regulated clinical research requires high-quality, or "sushi-grade," data, which can be obtained from EHRs if certain processes are applied and requirements met.

Levy

- Information from patient diagnosis, treatment, and treatment response should be aggregated and transformed to computable, standardized data for improved and more effective clinical decision support.
- EHR data quality issues may be mitigated through triangulation of multiple sources.
- Genome-directed cancer treatment is a driving-use case for learning cancer systems.

Buehler

- Data quality requirements depend on the purpose of those data.
- Public health surveillance systems must be prepared to take full advantage of the data influx resulting from implementation of Meaningful Use.
- Linking public health and direct health care services research through data will serve to strengthen the population-level approach to surveillance.

LaVenture

- Requirements for public health data quality vary by the specific program needs.
- Greater EHR use with improved standards and quality checks will increase the prevalence of better-quality data to improve care and public health.
- Incomplete records from EHRs with limited standards, specifications, and certification criteria create obstacles for the use of that data for surveillance.
- Value of data, and quality improvement, must be taught and encouraged as a standard of practice.
- A reliable bidirectional exchange of data with public health requires a shared responsibility for achieving high levels of data quality.

INTRODUCTION

Different data uses have different requirements and priorities. This chapter includes presentations and discussions focused on data uses and quality requirements from the perspectives of various stakeholders in the field. Mark Leenay, Chief Medical Officer and Senior Vice President at OptumHealth Care Solutions, discussed challenges and opportunities specific to practice management and the clinical care digital data utility. Rebecca Kush, Founder and the current President and CEO of Clinical Data Interchange Standards Consortium (CDISC), built on this topic in her discussion of data quality requirements, challenges, priorities and enabling standards/processes for the clinical research enterprise. Later, Mia Levy, Director of Cancer Clinical Informatics for the Vanderbilt-Ingram Cancer Center, detailed the case example of Vanderbilt's experience and successes in implementing a translational informatics data management system for cancer diagnosis, treatment, and care. James Buehler, Director of the Public Health Surveillance & Informatics Program Office at the Centers for Disease Control and Prevention (CDC), focused on data quality for public health surveillance at the national level, while Marty LaVenture, Director of the Office of Health Information Technology and e-Health at the Minnesota Department of Health, spoke to the local and state levels.

PRACTICE MANAGEMENT

In his discussion of the digital data utility and its role in clinical practice management, Mark Leenay emphasized the requirements necessary to enable sustainable private health information exchanges while ensuring data are connected, intelligent, and aligned. Actionable data at the point of care, increased data liquidity, and integration of data across the care continuum, as well as across different types of data, are all integral to incorporating digital health data into practice management.

While the quality of health data is important to their use, Leenay said, flow of data also plays a major role in supporting population management. Currently, data platforms are not integrated into routine care, rendering the flow of digital health information incomplete, and leaving the many different stakeholders managing care with only a partial view of the situation. Without a central repository of digital health information, from which each stakeholder is able to extract information to make decisions, this ineffective communication stream is difficult to rectify. The current lack of information fluidity, Leenay concluded, warrants continued efforts designed to bring data to the point of care for individuals.

In conjunction with the challenge of fluidity, identity resolution continues to be a barrier to providing integrated, longitudinal data. Without national member IDs, for both patients and providers, effective use of digital health data for practice management will continue to be a struggle. As an example of this challenge, Leenay cited that out of people using health care exchanges, it is predicted that 50 percent will be eligible for Medicaid at some point during the year. As these individuals presumably will alternate between a private exchange and Medicaid, integrating their data presents a challenge. Further complicating the issue, National Provider IDs (NPIs) are used inconsistently, which causes difficulties for data aggregation across provider and hospital groups.

Content within data systems, both administrative and clinical, presents additional challenges. Leenay suggested that 85 percent of the information in EHRs is administrative rather than clinical data. Administrative claims data typically are designed for fee-for-service billing as opposed to pay-for-performance. Historically, incentives have been designed to reward complexity of service; the more complex the service, the more the provider will be paid. However, as the system shifts to pay-for-performance, incentives will need to be structured so that physicians are incentivized to enter more clinical data in order to be reimbursed appropriately. Additionally, the limited link between claims data and clinical data, and provider resistance to efforts to forge that link, presents a challenge to supporting the sorts of analyses that require insight into both cost or utilization and clinical outcomes. Citing an area for potential short-term progress, Lennay mentioned that from a clinical data perspective, there is minimal use of national registries. Such registries could provide a way to look at clinical outcomes that are not necessarily as complex as EHRs. As a cautionary note, Lennay pointed out that from an administrative dataset perspective, migration from ICD-9 to ICD-10 will involve a transition from fewer data points to more, a complicated extrapolation that will be an ongoing challenge.

Lastly, Leenay emphasized, the data actually included in EHRs are often inconsistent and incomplete. However, in light of the changing health care environment, primarily the development of accountable care organizations (ACOs), data quality requirements are changing. He pointed out that ACOs represent an alignment of incentives for the collection of higher quality data, with greater completeness and accuracy, and the increased liquidity of this data.

In summary, Leenay underscored several priorities to improve integration of the digital data utility into clinical care moving forward: identity resolution, information exchange standards, registries, and attention to disparities. Identity resolution will be critical to increase the accuracy of digital record use for patient care; strategies to develop and improve current dataset systems must include a focus on standards and normalization to facilitate coordinated information exchange. Organizations and clinicians should make greater use of national registries. And given the current

DIGITAL HEALTH DATA USES 19

socioeconomic disparities in health care, it is important for stakeholders in the digital movement to guard against worsening such disparities through the digital divide.

CLINICAL RESEARCH

In her discussion of clinical research, Rebecca Kush emphasized that different types of analyses require different grades of data quality, likening the data quality requirements for clinical decisions and regulated research to "sushi-grade" data, or the highest quality available. As depicted in Figure 3-1, Kush laid out these requirements on a sliding scale, dependent

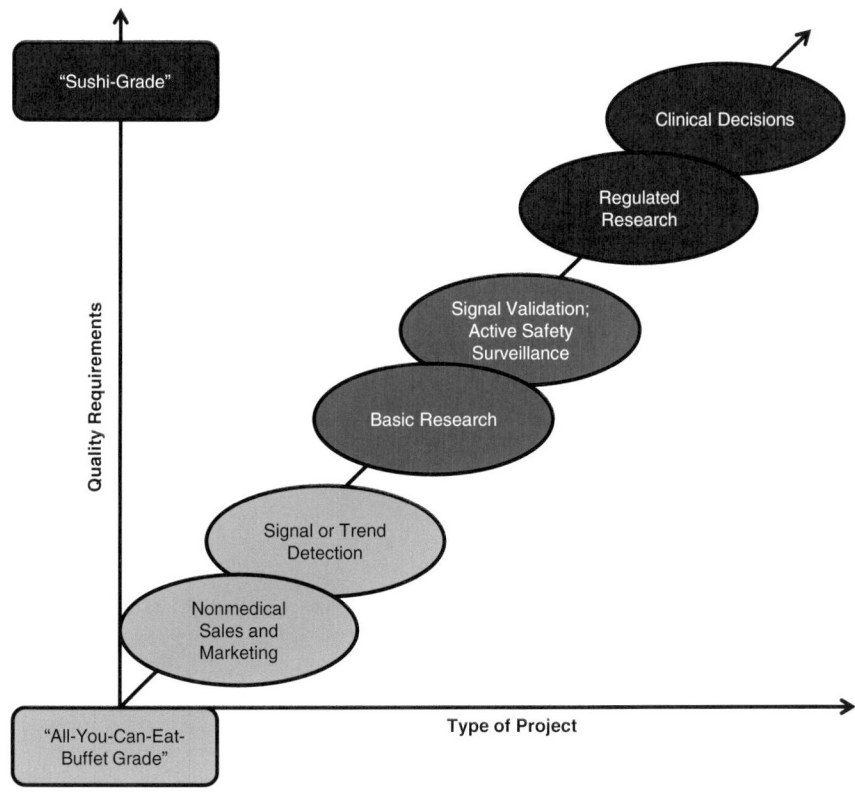

FIGURE 3-1 Spectrum of data quality requirements based on intended use.
SOURCE: Reprinted with permission from Rebecca Kush.

on the type of activities supported. Pointing to the extremes, she suggested that those projects investigating nonmedical sales and marketing have far different data quality requirements than those involving regulated research and clinical decisions.

Currently, Kush said, clinical research (especially regulated clinical research) presents a plethora of logistical challenges to clinical investigators. The average active study site has 3 or more disparate data entry systems; 50-60 percent of trials involve paper data collection on 3- or 4-part forms, while the remaining 40-50 percent of trials involve electronic data capture tools. Data are entered 4-7 times total on average, including 2-3 times by the clinicians or study coordinators. Thus, there is plenty of opportunity to introduce transcription errors. In addition, reporting an unexpected or serious adverse event does not fit into normal clinical care workflow and takes excessive time, so that researchers often refrain from doing so. Given these inefficiencies and labor-intensive procedures, Kush emphasized, most clinicians do one regulated clinical research study and no more. Further exacerbating the data quality issue, efforts to ensure that study data are clean can involve significant resources and financial consequences; depending on the point of the research process in which the error is identified, correction of a single error in the database can cost upward of $8,000.

However, promise lies in the growing industry appreciation of the power of standardization. Kush described CDISC's progress in this field through development of integration profiles with the capability to enable the extraction of a standardized, clinical research dataset (CDASH, Clinical Data Acquisition Standards Harmonization) from EHRs. The resulting interoperability specification (a set of standards) meets global regulations for collection of electronic research data and produces the minimum dataset needed on any clinical trial for regulated purposes. This combination of workflow enablers and standards has been used in safety reporting, regulatory reporting, and Phase 4 trials; and presents an opportunity to support research with EHRs and contribute to the process of research informing clinical decisions faster with higher quality information.

Kush then pointed to the Coalition Against Major Diseases (CAMD), an effort initiated by the Critical Path Institute (C-Path) to pool Alzheimer's-related trial data from multiple sources with the goal of generating better information from a larger, aggregated database. By standardizing this data into the CDISC format and then pooling it across sources, C-Path was able to create a database of more than 6,000 patients and has now made this database available to researchers around the world. A standard guide has been developed for researchers moving forward, so that they can collect Alzheimer's data in the CDISC format from the start and it can be easily compared with the current database. As such, this standardization effort has allowed researchers the capability to easily break out different cohorts and better identify trends in their patient populations in order to identify personalized treatments or to populations most likely to respond.

With CAMD as an exemplar of the opportunities available, Kush delineated priorities for clinical research to bring such successes to scale across the field. Data quality should be built into the clinical research system from the beginning, and those individuals involved in the research process (including site personnel, the project team, reviewers, and auditors) should be trained and educated to incorporate data quality measures, including standards for data collection, into their work. Data collection should be simplified with well-defined requirements for the necessary data set and standardized formats. Data should be handled only the minimum amount throughout the process, thereby reducing potential errors due to transcription or reentry. Additionally, Kush noted, data quality measures should be considered and incorporated throughout the postmarketing process.

In her final comments, Kush emphasized that greater standardization offers considerable promise for clinical research moving forward, particularly in leveraging EHRs for research. As exemplified by CAMD and similar efforts, standardization facilitates both data sharing and data aggregation, presenting the opportunity for groundbreaking research efforts to identify new treatments and therapies with larger, standardized datasets.

TRANSLATIONAL INFORMATICS

In her discussion of translational informatics, Mia Levy focused on her experience at the Vanderbilt-Ingram Cancer Center, where genome-directed cancer treatment is the focus of the Center's work. Currently, Levy noted, genomics is playing an ever more important role in the care of patients across the cancer continuum; cancer diagnosis, treatment selection, and care are all experiencing an era of genomics.

Traditionally, cancers have been categorized and treated according to the site of their origin and their histology. Now, the molecular subtypes of cancers are determining the course of care, and the molecular variance being discovered in these subtypes is vast. Levy noted that for those patients with characterized molecular subtypes, their mutations are considered actionable. Either an FDA-approved, standard-of-care therapy is available to treat the subtype of their cancer or a medication for their specific mutation is in the clinical research pipeline. However, in this genomic era, even patients for whom a mutation has not been identified are also considered to be actionable, in that they are spared from receiving ineffective, costly, and potentially harmful treatments. These developments hold great promise for the field of cancer treatment, but the process of implementing a system capable of processing and managing this information poses an entirely new range of challenges to those involved in translational informatics.

Reporting molecular diagnostic results in an EHR is typically unstructured and unwieldy she stated. Text is entered into a reporting template, and that form is then scanned and uploaded into the EHR as an image file, rendering it noncomputable. Another challenge associated with this type of reporting is the sheer amount of data to be reported. In her example, Levy highlighted that variance on 40 different mutations had to be reported at the same time. Not only does that require an increase in data points, but the complexity associated with this variance information must also be reflected in the system. Information must be reported in a way that is clinically useful for physicians, in order to help inform them of the findings' clinical significance. Levy emphasized that much of this information is actionable only through its ability to link a patient's results to clinical trial eligibility, and traditional reporting mechanisms do not possess this ability.

Levy noted that approaches to addressing these challenges are varied. Visualization of test results, complete with color coordination and coding, has proved very helpful at Vanderbilt, allowing researchers and clinicians to quickly scan information and identify positive findings. Findings are reported in a structured way, so that there is an entity, an attribute, and a value behind each piece of data. Moreover, information and results recorded in the EHR are linked directly to a database that provides information on the clinical significance of a patient's particular mutation variant, thereby identifying potential targeted therapies. Further guidance is provided through inclusion of relevant, summarized clinical trial literature, which links clinicians to full, PubMed sources should they need to see additional information on the significance of the trial to their patient's care. The data management system also links the EHR to a clinical trials database, providing clinicians with the means to identify relevant trial eligibility criteria. All of these strategies, Levy emphasized, offer promise for the effective and efficient incorporation of complex and varied digital data into the process of cancer care.

Levy finished her discussion by looking to the future, contemplating how to make systems like Vanderbilt's sustainable and scalable with respect to content generation as well as content dissemination. Aggregation of institutional data, she suggested, is critical for rendering the data clinically useful. Information from patient diagnosis, treatment, and treatment response should be aggregated and transformed to computable, standardized data for improved and more effective clinical decision support. Moreover, the records incorporated into this type of database should be combined with other data, including patient-reported outcomes as well as cost information, both of which would be beneficial to understanding treatment comparative effectiveness. Given the complexity of genome-directed cancer treatment and translational informatics on the whole, Levy underscored her experiences with the importance of triangulation of data from multiple sources to better approximate the probability of an event and use this as a basis for learning processes. EHR data can be useful for learning systems, but it must be of high quality and mitigated through triangulation of multiple resources.

SUPPORTING PUBLIC HEALTH AND SURVEILLANCE AT THE NATIONAL LEVEL

In the context of public health surveillance, data quality has varying definitions. As James Buehler of the CDC explained in his comments, quality requirements depend on the public health purpose the data are serving. For those working to prevent and contain specific diseases or adverse health events, the required data includes information about disease characteristics and severity, where and when it is occurring, its antecedents, its evolution over time, and its consequences. Moreover, public health professionals need data on those who are affected, individuals' risk factors and whether certain groups of people are affected more than others, outcomes, and disease susceptibility to treatment. All of this information, often generated by individuals' utilization of health care services, provides insight into what can be done to craft, target, and direct and redirect public health interventions. As such, public health surveillance is not simply about collecting information; it is about analyzing and using that data for a purpose, and that purpose can vary from disease surveillance, to situational awareness of a community's status, to local, sometimes individual, interventions. While the data-quality requirements vary for each of these different purposes, Buehler continued, some apply to the broad range of public health surveillance uses. The data should be complete, reliable, timely, and inexpensive, and they should provide accurate insights into the local surveillance context. In practice, it is often not possible for a surveillance system to achieve all of these desirable attributes, requiring balance of desirable and sometimes competing attributes to maximize utility and value.

In order to meet these requirements, current public health surveillance data sources and systems are becoming progressively more automated. Attention is increasingly directed toward integrating EHRs into both the reporting and feedback arms of surveillance, so that individuals' direct interactions with the health care system can serve as an additional source of electronic public health data. However, the process of moving this automation and integration forward faces a number of challenges Buehler noted, outlining several priorities for addressing those challenges. It is critical that public health surveillance systems are prepared to take full advantage of the data influx resulting from implementation of meaningful use, he said. The public health workforce likewise must be equipped to make the best use of this information, as it presents a great opportunity for more effective and efficient public health surveillance. Finally, he noted, linking public health and direct health care services research in this way will serve to strengthen the population-level approach to surveillance.

SUPPORTING PUBLIC HEALTH AND SURVEILLANCE AT THE LOCAL LEVEL

In line with Buehler's discussion of public health surveillance at the national level, Martin LaVenture shifted the focus to public health at the state and local (city and county) level. LaVenture reinforced the earlier assertion that necessary data quality attributes vary and depend on the context of the local public health activity. For example, timeliness is of particular importance for newborn screening, acute disease surveillance, and outbreaks, while completeness is especially critical for maintenance of immunization records. Accuracy is crucial for monitoring cancer clusters, while currency, comprehensiveness, and access to the primary data source all are relevant for public health surveillance and clinical decision support.

These quality characteristics all contribute to the usability of public health surveillance data today. Currently, surveillance data is collected from many sources, and health facilities increasingly are adopting EHRs for patient information management and decision support. However, frequent miscoding and mismapping of this information can result in loss of trust in both the data and the providers using those data; in which case the value of those data suffers. Moreover, the limited EHR standards and specifications and certification criteria lead to incomplete and invalid records, which create obstacles to efficient use of that data for clinical and disease surveillance purposes. This can lead to additional work by providers and public health officials and delay important public health intervention, prevention, and policy decisions.

In the face of these challenges, LaVenture said, the public health digital environment is changing. Greater EHR use with standards and quality checks built in will increase the prevalence of better quality data, thereby creating the opportunity for quality information exchange for care and public health and improved point-of-care decision support. To facilitate this progress, LaVenture proposed a number of priorities. Health information systems need to move beyond information management to rapid, accurate knowledge creation with support from public health information systems such as an immunization information system. The EHR certification process, he suggested, should include more comprehensive, structured content requirements for data quality, including thresholds at the point of capture, review, and exchange thus helping ensure higher-quality outputs for broader use. Standards for quality checks and improvement are needed to ensure updates and corrections can be completed quickly and propagation of errors to other settings can be minimized. LaVenture went on to suggest that health care professionals should be educated on the value of quality data to encourage further focus on and enthusiasm for high-quality data, and incentives should encourage use of this data to increase value and quality. Public health agencies need similar incentives and support to modernize state and local systems in order to enable bidirectional flow of this information. Additionally, LaVenture noted that better use of existing standards and adopting new standards for the content and quality of data will reduce variability and increase usability for multiple purposes, and continuous improvement of data sources will ensure that their output is of the highest quality possible. It is also critical that information generated from these sources, and the knowledge from its analysis, is brought back to the source, to foster continuous improvement at the source level. Finally, LaVenture concluded by emphasizing that continued innovation with the public health case in mind will lead to better-quality data and better surveillance through improved adoption, use, and exchange of health information.

4

Issues and Opportunities in the Emergence of Large Health-Related Datasets

---

KEY SPEAKER THEMES

Madigan

- Complexity of health information surpasses the ability of clinicians and current "evidence-based" models.
- Large health-related datasets can produce more accurate predictive models.
- Bias presents an enormous challenge to observational research but there are strategies to mitigate its impact.

McCall

- Understanding what works best for whom requires a nuanced understanding of cause and effect.
- Advances in mathematics, coupled with access to large datasets, have the potential to allow researchers to discover cause-effect relationships rather than correlations.
- Research should focus on insights rather than analytics in order to come up with causal structure rather than static answers.

INTRODUCTION

The emergence of large health-related datasets—from sources such as large health systems, payers, pharmacy benefit managers, etc.—have the potential to transform the clinical effectiveness research enterprise. Realizing the potential requires mathematical methods that handle the scale of data, as well as an appreciation of the biases and limitations inherent to each data source. David Madigan, Professor and Chair of the Department of Statistics at Columbia University, discussed the challenge of bias in large datasets, and strategies and methods to more appropriately address bias in observational clinical outcomes research. Carol McCall, Chief Strategy Officer at GNS Healthcare, focused on new mathematical approaches that allow nuanced insights to be derived from large datasets.

THE CHALLENGE OF BIAS IN LARGE HEALTH-RELATED DATASETS

David Madigan began his presentation by focusing on the current clinical decision framework, which revolves around evidence-based medicine and clinical judgment. He told the story of a cardiologist deciding whether or not a patient should receive angioplasty. Using a risk assessment algorithm from the Framingham study, the doctor assigned a 10-year risk of developing coronary heart disease using the following variables: age, total cholesterol, smoking, high-density lipoprotein (HDL), and blood pressure. According to Madigan, this is evidence-based medicine in 2012. A multitude of other health related data—other lab results, family history, medication, other health issues—is ignored in this analysis. This is where, ideally, clinical judgment comes in. The cardiologist should use the evidence-based recommendation, coupled with the other variables, to make an appropriate decision. Madigan argued that in the face of this much information it is infeasible for a human being to do optimal decision making.

With the right statistical techniques, however, large health-related datasets can begin to answer these questions. Madigan cited the work of the Observational Medical Outcomes Partnership (OMOP), which has medical records for roughly 200 million individuals. Within this database, he speculated, there might be 30,000 individuals like the patient described above. This information can be used to make inferences about the course of care more precisely than those made by physicians. At its heart, Madigan stated, these are issues of predictive modeling. The way that "big data" can help improve care is by aiding the development of good predictive models.

According to Madigan, the data for these types of analyses exist. There are several databases with large quantities of patient-level data. The limitation is that, currently, there are no satisfactory methodologies to build

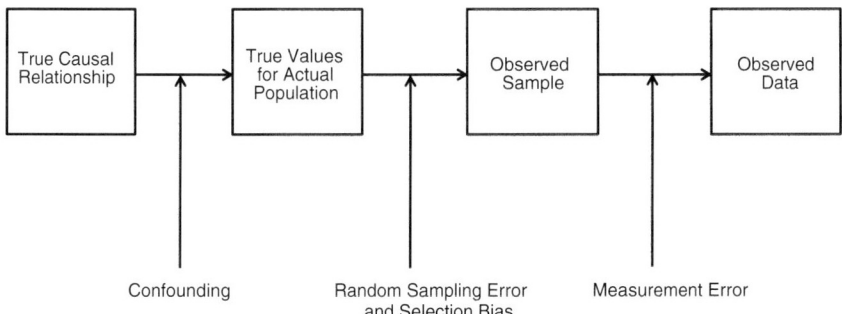

FIGURE 4-1 Sources of bias in clinical datasets.
SOURCE: Reprinted with permission from Phillips, 2003.

reliable predictive models. One challenge is the inherent bias of the data being used. Madigan laid out the various stages in the data collection and research process at which bias can be introduced into a data set (Figure 4-1).

Bias alone is not the problem. In fact, it is unavoidable. The larger problem is that current observational research with large datasets does not acknowledge the limitations that bias places on results. Madigan noted that, generally, the issues of bias and measurement error are only paid lip service in the peer-reviewed literature for observational clinical outcomes research. Articles will often state potential limitations, but fail to discuss the implications. There are profound data quality issues when using large observational datasets and, according to Madigan, the current practice for observational research does little about it.

To demonstrate the consequence of bias he presented some data from the OMOP database. OMOP researchers ran self-controlled case series analysis for a variety of drugs across each of the 10 component OMOP databases. The results demonstrated extreme heterogeneity. For 20 of the 50 drug-event pairs studies, the drug-event relationship went from being statistically significant in the positive direction to statistically significant in the negative direction depending on which database was used. This heterogeneity has profound implications for the generalizability of published outcomes research.

Madigan concluded his presentation by focusing on strategies that confront these challenges of bias and data quality. One critical strategy is sensitivity analysis. He acknowledged that sound statistical methods and software for sensitivity analysis currently exist. These methods look at sources of biases and run various "what-if" scenarios to give a sense of how robust findings are. He suggested that sensitivity analysis ought to be an absolute requirement for the publication of observational studies.

The other strategy to improve the quality and utility of retrospective outcomes research is to establish operating characteristics of observational studies. Madigan argued that currently there is no good understanding of the quality and reliability of this type of research. For example, if a study arrives at a certain relative risk, how close is that relevant risk to the truth if it were to be reproduced with different data? Similarly, when studies report 95 percent confidence intervals, how close are those to the truth? Madigan noted that OMOP researchers have found that across databases, reported 95 percent confidence intervals often have only roughly 50 percent coverage. There is a need, he stressed, to study this science empirically in order to get a handle on how well it actually works and how likely the results are to be the truth.

MOVING FROM ANALYTICS TO INSIGHTS

Carol McCall posed that the principal challenge in health care today is the ability to create a deep and dynamic understanding of what works best for whom. She noted that while there are currently many areas of redesign and improvement in health care—aligning business models, transforming care models, building infrastructure—all of these changes implicitly assume that there is access to evidence and an understanding of what works for whom. The sustainability of all of these efforts demands something new: a nuanced understanding of cause and effect in health care.

According to McCall, three developments have made it possible to analyze vast amounts of data to generate actionable medical evidence. The first is Moore's law, the doubling of computing capacity approximately every 2 years, which gave rise to big data and big-data technologies. The second is that health care data is becoming much more liquid. The third, which she noted as the lynchpin, is a revolution in mathematics, led by Judea Pearl, which has mathematized causality, opening a paradigm shift in analytics. Previously, the problem with big data was that the bigger it got, the more correlations were found. McCall stressed that correlation is a truism. Data is correlated, always higher or lower, but it always exists, and it is *not* the same as causation. This new calculus of causality, however, allows researchers to discover cause-effect relationships and generate evidence from big data (Pearl, 2009).

The fundamental difference of this type of approach is that it focuses on insights rather than analytics. Through these types of mathematical methods, she notes, researchers are left with causal structure rather than a static answer. This structure can be interrogated to answer a variety of important questions such as what data is needed to resolve existing uncertainty, an insight that can guide next data investments and be used to tailor research strategies. Furthermore, this type of structure allows researchers to run counterfactuals, interrogate and investigate much more quickly, and go beyond situations where they already know the answer. This ability to make predictions and quickly assess results is at the core of a learning health system. Clinicians and researchers can predict an outcome, observe what happens, compare it against experience, and adjust future care protocols in response. And this can all happen rapidly.

With the mathematical methods in place, McCall noted, the priorities for big data analytics and evidence generation are shifting. Since mathematics can be scaled to any level and performed on any data set, the challenge now is finding data sources that are comprehensive and up to date. She underscored the need to link and share data from a variety of sources, such as pharmaceutical companies, hospitals, pharmaceutical benefit managers and payers. With data coming from several sources, there is also the need to understand context, and metadata take on an added importance.

REFERENCES

Pearl, J. 2009. *Causality: Models, reasoning and inference.* New York: Cambridge University Press.

Phillips, C. V. 2003. Quantifying and reporting uncertainty from systematic errors. *Epidemiology* 14(4):459-466.

5

Innovations Emerging in the Clinical Data Utility

KEY SPEAKER THEMES

Elmore and Platt

- Distributed data queries can provide the foundation of a learning health system.
- Advantages of distributed data networks include data accuracy, timeliness, flexibility, and sustainability.
- Distributed queries facilitate asking questions of large datasets in ways that are HIPAA-compliant and maintain local context.

Chute

- Data normalization and harmonization are critical to ensuring effective and accurate secondary use.
- There are multiple approaches to data normalization, but a hybrid approach of new systems standardizing from inception and legacy systems transforming over time is most feasible.
- Clinical element models, together with value sets, present opportunity for normalization in a way that maintains the context and provenance of the data.
- Value-set management is a major component of normalization, and terminology service; a national repository of value sets is one suggested approach to handling this challenge.

> **Kheterpal**
> - Modern health care challenges, such as chronic disease, require comprehensive, longitudinal information to support team care.
> - Blindfolded record linkage, such as using hashes, offer many advantages to better link data between sources while maintaining privacy.

INTRODUCTION

In order to make optimal use of the digital health data utility, novel and innovative approaches will have to be developed. These innovations include learning from large sets of data while dealing with the risk associated with physical aggregation, coping with incomplete standardization of data, and linking data from diverse sources without the use of universal identifiers. Richard Elmore, Coordinator of Query Health at the Office of the National Coordinator for Health Information Technology, and Richard Platt, Chair of Population Medicine at Harvard Medical School and Harvard Pilgrim Health Care Institute, discussed the specific case of distributed data queries. Christopher Chute, Professor of Medical Informatics at the Mayo Clinic, elaborated on challenges and opportunities associated with data harmonization and normalization. Vik Kheterpal, Principal at CareEvolution, focused on data linkage between sources.

DISTRIBUTED QUERIES

In their discussion of distributed queries, Richard Elmore and Richard Platt covered the broad definition and qualities of such queries, and provided specific examples of these queries in action. Distributed queries allow querying of data from multiple partners without having to physically aggregate data in one central repository; a query is sent to all partners, and each participant runs this query internally and returns summary results individually. Some example use cases for distributed population queries include population measures related to disease outbreaks, postmarket surveillance, prevention, quality, and performance. The advantages of this model, Elmore emphasized, are myriad. A distributed query approach allows data partners to maintain HIPAA-mandated, contractual control of their protected health information (PHI), and it facilitates data validity by ensuring that results are returned by local content experts, those most familiar with and understanding of the data and their interpretation. The distributed data environment also supports data accuracy, timeliness, flexibility, and sustainability.

Despite their many advantages, distributed queries also face a number of data quality challenges. Complications in integrating results from several data sources due to a lack of standards were cited as an example. But, Elmore said, pathbreaking work is under way to address this problem. Difficulty in striking a balance between clinical intuitiveness and computability when expressing a query is another challenge. Moreover, once a query is formulated, the lack of semantic equivalency and standards to express clinical concepts among data systems must be addressed. Additionally, there is no cultivated standard value set, clinicians in the same practice often code differently, and each organization has its own established value sets. Furthermore, within those value sets, data are often missing, so completeness also presents a challenge to distributed queries.

Despite the obstacles inherent to such queries, several examples, across many domains, are ongoing and have achieved great success. Platt described Mini-Sentinel, an FDA-sponsored pilot initiative that has created a distributed dataset that includes data on 126 million people at 17 data partners to support active safety surveillance of medical products. The FDA now routinely uses the system.

Platt cited an example of a query dealing with drugs for smoking cessation, addressing concern that a certain drug increased risk of negative cardiac outcomes. Within 3 days of receiving FDA's intent to query the network, Mini-Sentinel returned its first report on the results, including information on 300 million person years of experience. While the speed and scope of the query result were impressive, Platt noted that it had several associated limitations. These included that it was intended to be a quick look, not a final answer; that the result did not exclude excess risk; and that recorded exposures may have been missing or included a misclassified indication. Moreover, the cohort may have been unrepresentative, outcomes may have been misclassified, and there was a potential for residual confounding due to disparate smoking intensities or comorbidities. Nonetheless, with the right clarification on the query itself, specifications on the cohort of interest, and selection of diagnosis codes, the network was able to rapidly query hundreds of millions of people's worth of data without transferring any institution's PHI.

Another query focused on a comparison of individuals who had experienced a stroke or transient ischemic attack (TIA) and previously received one of two different types of platelet antagonists. Treatment with one of the platelet antagonists was counter-indicated for individuals who had previously had a stroke or TIA; Mini-Sentinel determined that half as many individuals received the counter-indicated drug following stroke or TIA compared to those individuals receiving the comparison drug. The limitations inherent to this query included that the ICD-9 codes used for TIA and stroke were not validated in Mini-Sentinel, and that the longest look back for stroke or TIA events was 1 year, so that patients who experienced an event earlier than 1 year prior were missed.

In both of these examples, it was possible to get very quick information that provided guidance that FDA found to be useful in determining how much urgency should be attached to a specific question, while also helping to develop next steps. Along these lines, Query Health, an ONC-sponsored initiative, is working with many partners to develop standards for distributed data queries. As Elmore emphasized, the idea is to send questions to voluntary, collaborative networks, whose varied data sources may range from EHRs, to health information exchanges (HIEs), to other clinical records. These queries have the potential to dramatically cut cycle time on population questions, from years to days, and thereby, Elmore said, are critical to ONC's strategy to bend the curve toward transformed health, and will play a foundational role in the digital infrastructure for a learning health system, focusing on the patient and patient populations, while ensuring privacy and trust.

DATA HARMONIZATION AND NORMALIZATION

In his comments on data harmonization and normalization, Christopher Chute stressed that data from patient encounters must be comparable and consistent in order to provide knowledge and insights to inform future care decisions. This normalization is also necessary for big-data approaches to queries. However, most clinical data in the United States, even within institutions, are heterogeneous, which presents a major challenge for harmonization efforts. ONC's initiation of Meaningful Use is mitigating this challenge, but more work is needed.

Data normalization, Chute said, comes in two varieties: clinical data normalization of structured information, and processing of unstructured natural language. Moreover, three potential approaches to instituting this normalization exist. The first approach is for all generators of data, including lab systems, departmental systems, physician entry systems, to normalize their data at the source. Given the institutional effort necessary to realize this approach, it is not realistic in the short term. The second approach places all hopes for normalization in transformation and mapping on the back end of data systems; this approach sometimes works, but often is associated with ambiguous meanings and other transformation difficulties. Lastly, the third and most promising method is a hybrid approach, in which new systems begin by normalizing their data at the source, while established systems implement standard normalization protocols like meaningful use and data from legacy systems are transformed.

In discussing these approaches, Chute emphasized, it is important to comprehend fully the definition of normalization, as it has both syntactic and semantic meanings. Syntactic normalization is highly mechanical and involves correction of malformed messages. An example of such work is the Health Open Source Software pipeline created by Regenstrief Institute, which is capable of this type of syntactic normalization. On the other hand, semantic normalization typically involves vocabulary and concept mapping.

Both types of normalization assume that there is a normal form to target, yet extant national and international standards do not fully specify that target. Many standards exist, but, Chute said, they do not specify what is needed. The current standards and specifications of HIE and messaging are narrow, and do not look at the full representational problems of clinical data, so that efforts to meet the standards fall short on those fronts. Additionally, while there is tension on this point, machine readable, rather than human readable, standard representation is necessary for large-scale inferencing and secondary use.

Having elaborated on the definition and current characteristics of normalization, Chute turned to describing current efforts undertaken by ONC's Strategic Health IT Advanced Research Projects (SHARP) Program, specifically SHARPn, whose major focus is on normalizing and standardizing data. SHARPn is approaching data normalization through clinical element model (CEM) structures, which are a basis for retaining consistent meaning for data when they are exchanged between heterogeneous computer systems or when clinical data are referenced in decision support logic or other modalities of secondary use. CEMs include the context and provenance of data, for example a patient's position and body location will be recorded alongside his or her blood pressure reading.

This promising model has generated an international consortium, the Clinical Information Model Initiative (CIMI), which brings together a variety of efforts focused on CEMs. When comparing the resulting CEMs between different participating partners, it becomes clear that different secondary uses require different metadata, which raises the question of what structured information should be incorporated into these models. By binding value sets to CEMs, Chute suggested, it is possible to effectively institute semantic normalization. Ideally, all collaborating groups would implement the same value sets and they would be drawn from "standard vocabularies" like LOINC and SNOMED. However, it is likely that many value sets would have to be bound to these CEMs in order to truly have interoperability and a comparable and consistent representation of clinical data. Value-set management, therefore, is a major component of normalization, and terminology services and a national repository of value sets managed by the National Library of Medicine is one suggested approach to handling this challenge. Local codes would have to map to the major value sets, and the process of semantic mapping from local codes to "standard" codes, Chute emphasized, surely would be labor intensive. This underscores the critical importance of tagging data at the local level, so that those who best understand the data's significance are the individuals determining its codes.

DATA LINKAGE

Vik Kheterpal began by emphasizing chronic disease as the dominant problem in health care as a way to highlight the challenges associated with data linkage. Chronic diseases are the principal cause of disability and health services utilization, and account for 78 percent of health care expenditures. Care for these conditions necessitates teamwork and coordination between multiple caregivers, and this team-based care requires data exchange, interoperability, and management over a patient's extended care timeline. The data must be longitudinal and its management must be coordinated in order to ensure that clinicians are able to view the patient's condition across time before making clinical decisions. This level of coordination, Kheterpal suggested, offers the opportunity to reduce costs, improve outcomes, and reduce care fragmentation.

In working toward this more interoperable vision of data exchange, it is important that the current focus on EHRs be broadened, Kheterpal suggested. He emphasized the need to focus not on the technology, but what can be done with it. For example, EHRs are necessary to facilitate exchange, but they are not sufficient to accrue transformational systemic value. Rather than simply digitizing the data contained in paper records, emphasis should be placed on improving data visualization, and leveraging the power of large datasets for extrapolation. The strategy also must address health care specific challenges, including false positives, lack of uniform identifiers, privacy regulations, dirty data, and the multitude of data sources.

Kheterpal highlighted that data linkage is a major challenge to integrating data from different sources and to providing longitudinal data on patients in order to assess downstream outcomes and get a complete picture. To confront these challenges, Kheterpal said, blindfolded record linkage holds much promise. This method of linking data allows for secure, one-way hash transformations so that records can be linked without any party having to reveal identifying information about any of the subjects. Its advantages are numerous in that it maintains patient privacy, is already viable and in production, and can process large population sets. Moreover, Kheterpal said, current health data efforts can easily be adapted to include it. Employing this strategy for linking data can decrease duplicity and provide a longitudinal view of the patient's care history, two of the major challenges to optimizing learning from large datasets.

To close, Kheterpal offered several recommendations to move the field forward. Increased utilization of distributed blindfolded linkage pilots will provide greater evidence on their fitness to address the challenges at hand. Research into the scale of overlap and missed signal problems associated with systems that do not link records stratified across disease states will help to make the case for improved record linkage. Lastly, Kheterpal suggested development of a stratification model that matches a proposed research question with necessary data types could improve the accuracy and relevance of data linkage efforts.

6

Strategies Going Forward

During the final session of the workshop individual participants reflected on the day's presentations and discussions and discussed actions they felt were important to progress in the areas discussed. The suggestions made by individual participants covered six broad thematic areas: improving awareness and gap assessment of existing data sources; improving the quality, patient orientation, and utility of data input; improving the access, tools, and capacity for data analysis; ramping up the involvement and engagement of the patients and the public for improved clinical data; building a clinical data learning utility; and developing clarity on the governance needed.

CURRENT DATA SOURCES: BETTER AWARENESS AND ASSESSMENT

A number of speakers raised the issue of the need for a better understanding of what data sources exist, their characteristics, their relationships to each other, and the implications of these details on the uses of the data (see Chapters 2-5).

Resource mapping. Discussion during the final session yielded several suggestions from individual attendees on how to work toward getting a better understanding of digital health data sources. Assembling a taxonomy of digital health data sources with descriptors to better understand what sources are out there and their specific characteristics was suggested by a few participants as a potential first step toward this goal.

Utility mapping. It was suggested that the mapping process should also include not just taxonomy and inventory of data sources, but assessment of how high-priority questions and issues map to existing sources and methods, including annotation of sources used in research studies.

DATA INPUT: IMPROVE PATIENT ORIENTATION, QUALITY, AND UTILITY

As emphasized in *Crossing the Quality Chasm* in 2001, patient-centered care has been highlighted as a central component of quality health care (IOM, 2001). Extending this notion to digital health information was a frequent theme in workshop discussions.

Information patients care about. Several participants and speakers emphasized collecting information that patients care about, and including information on wellness and productivity, as a first step toward this goal. Similarly, increasing the inclusion of patient-reported information in the digital health data utility was highlighted as a priority. Development, validation, and encouragement of the use of patient-reported preferences, symptoms, care-process measures, and outcomes were called out as potential important components of this strategy.

Usability. Improving the usability of health and biomedical information technology and prioritizing information collection were strategies suggested to minimize the burden imposed on data collectors. Identifying and eliminating the collection of low-value data, as well as automating data collection, whenever appropriate, were suggested as potential approaches.

Contextual tagging. Maintenance of the provenance and context of the data was also highlighted as an important issue, particularly when data is used for a purpose other than that for which it was collected. The use of metadata tagging and strategies to enable access to full original context (e.g., on place, time, person/SES) were called out as potential approaches.

Core elements. In order to make progress on the goal of improving data quality, the development of more standardized digital health data definitions and representations was highlighted for attention. In particular, several participants emphasized the need for development of a set of core minimum standardized data elements to provide timely essential information on cost, quality, and health status and trends, available across institutions and geographic areas and designed to harmonize funder data set requirements. Some participants felt that inclusion of these core elements as part of the certification process was an effective way to further progress.

DATA ANALYSIS: IMPROVE ACCESS, TOOLS, AND CAPACITY

Only through analysis and use of digital health data will its full potential be realized (IOM, 2012). Improving the analytic tools and capacity necessary for learning were common themes in workshop discussions.

Toolsets. Specifically, the creation of toolsets that would expand access to tools and applications beyond the traditional research community and open opportunities for analysis and learning was cited as a potential approach with some precedence in other areas of science.

Curation. Strategies and methods to curate data sources in an ongoing way were also suggested. The need for better metrics to measure data quality and utility, in context-appropriate ways, was also discussed. Some participants suggested that these metrics could focus on the impact of information collection and input processes on the data; for example, data collection in the course of routine care through an EHR versus as part of a clinical trial.

Data integration. Several participants asserted that putting patients at the center of digital health data also included facilitating the integration of their data across the several facets of health, including with public health information and other sources, some of which may be external to health care. Strategies for data integration, in particular, including public health data, were suggested as a necessary first step toward this goal. A related concept of triangulating several data sources to improve predictive accuracy was also mentioned by several speakers as an important advantage to having large amounts of diverse data.

PUBLIC AND PATIENT ENGAGEMENT: RAMP UP INVOLVEMENT

Many participants stressed that successfully engaging stakeholders is crucial for fully realizing the learning and improvement potential of digital health data. Whether a data donor, collector, or user, a patient, clinician, public health official, or researcher, all stakeholders have unique, and changing, roles to play.

Patient voice. Drawing further from the notion of collecting and including information patients care about, many participants cited the need for a strong strategy for building the capacity for direct patient engagement. Specific approaches included the development and refinement of portals, and the inclusion of patient preferences and other patient-sourced data.

Trust. Building trust among stakeholders was a common denominator in issues identified to take advantage of expanding capacity for continuously learning health care. Several discussants noted that in order to create and nurture this trust, stakeholders must feel that their participation in data collection and use processes are respectful of their efforts, their privacy, and responsive to their needs.

Regulatory reform. Development of mutual understandings of expectations for confidentiality, privacy, and security were highlighted as key to building and maintaining strong stakeholder support in the rapidly evolving environment of social media, increased availability of information online, and the growing integration of genomics into clinical care and diagnostics.

Presentation. Increasing the usefulness of data to patients, and other stakeholders, through the use of user-appropriate data presentation techniques, including visualization, was suggested by several workshop participants.

Health literacy. A few participants cautioned that efforts to improve understanding through raising awareness and targeted strategies at different health literacy levels will be necessary to facilitate these discussions.

Culture of participation. Given this changing environment, the suggestion was made to empower potential data donors (notably patients) with the option and ability to donate their information for use. Along similar lines, the idea of studying the benefits and risks of patient-requested portable identifiers was suggested as a way to make progress on the issue of identity resolution and data linkage, and a first step toward developing a strategy for their development and application.

BUILDING A CLINICAL DATA LEARNING UTILITY

Throughout workshop presentations and discussions, some speakers and participants stressed the need to harness the potential for learning from the digital health data utility. The challenges and opportunities afforded by the increasing scale of data available for learning informed many of these discussions.

Innovative methods. The development of methods using EHRs as a data source and performing observational studies on big data were highlighted as specific needs. In particular, the development, validation, and use of predictive models to inform health-data uses, including risk interpretation by individuals, was singled out as holding great promise. Noting that most digital health data is in unstructured formats, the potential for learning from this data through natural language processing (e.g., IBM's Watson) was highlighted by several workshop participants. An emphasis on the need for the development and application of reasoning and inference tools was highlighted as a potential priority going forward.

Distributed approaches. Given the importance of privacy and security in the collection and use of patient health data, presentations and discussions frequently touched on the advantages of distributed data approaches and the need to further develop and pilot the policies, analytic methods, and technologies associated with their use.

Engaging bias. Several challenges and barriers to learning from the digital health data utility were cited, including uncertainty about the completeness and reliability of many data sources, as well as the presence of multiple forms of bias. The need for detailed expert assessments of the implications of bias on analyses, as well as in the new context of the very large datasets now emerging, was suggested by several workshop participants.

Core elements. The identification and application of a set of minimum data elements to provide information on cost, quality, health status, and health trends was suggested, by several discussants, as a critical component to accelerating progress on learning from the health data utility. Reform of regulatory frameworks to encourage structured collection, assessment, and use of routinely collected data, in order to facilitate and support this learning, was highlighted by some participants as an important first step.

CLARITY ON GOVERNANCE

Greater clarity on governance, both in terms of what it would look like and the issues for engagement, specifically in terms of access and sustainability, was a theme echoed in many workshop discussions.

Domains. Some participants pointed to a need to identify key domains for which governance structures are necessary to accelerate the evolution of the digital data utility, and begin to catalyze their engagement.

Access and ownership. Suggested approaches to ensuring participation included enabling broader access to data sources and ensuring that the flow of information is multidirectional. This democratization of roles could facilitate the engagement of the issue of data ownership, broaden sources of input, exhibit the potential of information use to meet stakeholder needs, and demonstrate the value of the collection and use of the data.

Business model. There is a need for a better understanding of both the costs and benefits associated with the uses of digital health data for learning and continuous improvement. Quantitative and qualitative approaches to insights on how information might be leveraged to increase health benefits and minimize associated costs from the perspectives of the many diverse stakeholders were highlighted by some participants as an important first step on this count. Additionally, the application of analytics for patient panel management and to support pay for performance payment initiatives such as ACOs were cited by individual participants as examples of areas of promise for establishing sustainable efforts.

REFERENCES

IOM (Institute of Medicine). 2001. *Crossing the quality chasm: A new health system for the 21st century*. Washington, DC: National Academy Press.

IOM. 2012. *Best care at lower cost: The path to continuously learning health care in America*. Washington, DC: The National Academies Press.

Appendix A

Speaker Biographies

James W. Buehler, MD, is the director of the Public Health Surveillance & Informatics Program Office (proposed) at the Centers for Disease Control and Prevention (CDC). Dr. Buehler has more than 30 years of experience in the field of medical epidemiology, serving from 1981 to 2002 as a commissioned officer in the U.S. Public Health Service at CDC, where he worked in the areas of general field epidemiology, maternal and child health, HIV/AIDS, and, for a brief period in 2001, anthrax. In 2002, Dr. Buehler joined the epidemiology department of the Rollins School of Public Health at Emory University, where he held the position of research professor. In 2009, he returned to CDC to contribute to the surveillance of pandemic influenza, and in 2010, he became the founding director of CDC's Public Health Surveillance Program Office. Dr. Buehler has devoted much of his career to the field of public health surveillance. As a member of the Emory faculty, Dr. Buehler's research interests centered on improving public health surveillance and emergency preparedness capacities and on advancing the relatively new field of public health systems research. While at Emory, he served as a consultant to epidemiology and emergency preparedness programs at the Division of Public Health of the Georgia Department of Human Resources. In 2006-2008, he served as the public health representative on the Georgia Health Information Technology and Transparency Advisory Board, where he focused on strengthening linkages between public health and health care through advances in health information technologies. Dr. Buehler obtained his bachelor's degree in biochemistry from the University of California, Berkeley, and his doctor of medicine degree from the University of California, San Francisco. He completed residency training in pediatrics at the University of Oregon Health Sciences Center in Portland and in preventive medicine at CDC. He is a fellow of the American Academy of Pediatrics and is board-certified in pediatrics and preventive medicine.

Christopher G. Chute, MD, DrPH, received his undergraduate and medical training at Brown University, completed his internal medicine residency at Dartmouth, and completed doctoral training in epidemiology at Harvard. He is board-certified in internal medicine, and is a fellow of the American College of Physicians, the American College of Epidemiology, and the American College of Medical Informatics. He became founding chair of biomedical informatics at Mayo in 1988, stepping down after 20 years in that role. He is now professor of medical informatics, and is principal investigator (PI) on a large portfolio of research, including the Department of Health and Human Services (HHS)/Office of the National Coordinator (ONC) SHARP (Strategic Health IT Advanced Research Projects) on Secondary EHR Data Use; the ONC Beacon Community (Co-PI); the LexGrid projects; Mayo's CTSA Informatics; Mayo's Cancer Center Informatics, including caBIG; and several National Institutes of Health (NIH) grants, including one of the eMERGE centers from the National Human Genome Research Institute. Dr. Chute serves as vice chair of the Mayo Clinic Data Governance for Health Information Technology Standards, and on Mayo's Enterprise IT Oversight Committee. He is presently chair, ISO Health Informatics Technical Committee (ISO TC215), and chairs the World Health Organization ICD-11 Revision. He also serves on the Health Information Technology Standards Committee for the Office of the National Coordinator in HHS, and the HL7 Advisory Board. His recently held positions include chair of the biomedical computing and health informatics study section at NIH; chair of the board of the HL7/FDA/NCI/CDISC BRIDG project; member of the board of the Clinical Data Interchange Standards Consortium; American National Standards Institute Health Information Standards Technology Panel (HISTP) board member; chair of the U.S. delegation to ISO TC215 for Health Informatics; Convener of Healthcare Concept Representation WG3 within the (TC215); co-chair of the HL7 Vocabulary Committee; chair of the International Medical Informatics Association WG6 on Medical Concept Representation; American Medical Informatics Association board member, and multiple other NIH biomedical informatics study sections as chair or member.

Rich Elmore is the Office of the National Coordinator's (ONC's) leader for Query Health, an ONC-sponsored initiative to establish standards and services for distributed population queries of electronic health records. He is on a leave of absence from health care technology provider Allscripts, where as vice president, strategic initiatives, he managed exploration and execution of acquisitions and strategic partnerships, and prior to that ran the Allscripts Provider Analytics business. He had a long career at IDX where he ran the Flowcast Hospital business and prior to that was vice president of product development for IDX Flowcast. Mr. Elmore was the communications workgroup leader for the ONC's Direct Project. He was a charter member of the interoperability workgroup for the Certification Commission for Healthcare Information Technology. Mr. Elmore has degrees from Dartmouth College (BA) and New School University (MA, economics). He is on the board of directors for Patient Engagement Systems, a chronic disease technology company, and serves as vice chair on the board of directors for the King Street Center, serving kids in need and their families in Burlington, Vermont.

Doug Fridsma, MD, PhD, is the director of the Office of Standards and Interoperability and the acting chief scientist in the Office of the National Coordinator for Health Information Technology (ONC). Prior to arriving at ONC, Dr. Fridsma was on the teaching staff in the department of biomedical informatics at Arizona State University and had a clinical practice at Mayo Clinic, Scottsdale. Dr. Fridsma completed his medical training at the University of Michigan in 1990, and his PhD in biomedical informatics from Stanford University in 2003. In his role at ONC, Dr. Fridsma is responsible for the Nationwide Health Information Network, the Federal Health Architecture, the EHR certification programs, and other initiatives focused on promoting interoperable health information exchange. He served on the Clinical Data Interchange Standards Consortium board of directors from 2005 to 2008, and was appointed to the Health IT Standards Committee in 2009. He resigned from the HIT Standards Committee after he joined ONC, and recently became a board member of HL7.

James Allen Heywood is the co-founder and chairman of PatientsLikeMe. A Massachusetts Institute of Technology engineer, Mr. Heywood entered the field of translational research and medicine when his brother Stephen was diagnosed with amyotrophic lateral sclerosis (ALS) in 1998 at the age of 29. With experience in design, information technology, systems modeling, neuroscience, and industrial engineering, Mr. Heywood brings a unique perspective to drug discovery and medicine. The scientific and business innovations he developed at the ALS Therapy Development Institute (TDI) and PatientsLikeMe have been transforming the intersection of biotechnology and pharmaceutical development, personalized medicine, and patient care. Heywood is the chairman of PatientsLikeMe, where he provides the scientific vision and architecture for its patient-centered medical platform. He co-founded the company in 2005 with his youngest brother, Benjamin, and his friend Jeff Cole. Named one of "15 companies that will change the world" by *CNNMoney*, PatientsLikeMe is a personalized research and peer care platform that allows patients to share in-depth information on treatments, symptoms, and outcomes. This novel open model allows clinicians, providers, and the pharmaceutical industry to better understand diseases and the patient experience. Patients improve their care and actively partner with industry to accelerate and influence the development of new treatments and biomarkers. In 1999, shortly after Stephen was diagnosed, Mr. Heywood founded the ALS TDI, the world's first nonprofit biotechnology company, where he served as CEO until 2007. Pioneering an open research model and an industrialized therapeutic validation process, Mr. Heywood led ALS TDI to become the world's largest and most comprehensive ALS research program. The comprehensive in vivo validation program Mr. Heywood developed was unable to replicate any of the published preclinical studies of the field that led to human trials, calling into question the standards that allowed many drugs to be tested on patients. In 2009, Mr. Heywood and a small group of thought leaders founded HealthDataRights.org, an organization that asserts a new patient's right to access a copy of all of his or her medical data in a computable form. Mr. Heywood is a published author, frequent speaker, media pundit, and active investment advisor. He speaks at business, government, and academic conferences around the world, including TEDMED, the Milken Global Conference, Health 2.0, Gov 2.0, Personal Democracy Forum, Institute of Medicine workshops, and the National Institutes of Health. Mr. Heywood is a member of the Centers for Disease Control and Prevention's National Biosurveillance Advisory Subcommittee, and has testified on privacy and social policy before the Department of Health and Human Services and the Food and Drug Administration. Mr. Heywood's work has been profiled in the *New Yorker*, *New York Times* magazine, *BusinessWeek*, *60 Minutes*, *CBS Evening News*, NPR, *Science*, and *Nature*. In 2009, he was chosen for WIRED magazine's "Smart List" and *Fast Company*'s "10 Most Creative People in Healthcare." Mr. Heywood and his brother Stephen were the subjects of Pulitzer Prize–winner Jonathan Wiener's biography *His Brother's Keeper* and the Sundance Award–winning documentary *So Much So Fast*.

Vik Kheterpal, MD, is a principal at CareEvolution, Inc., a leading provider of secure interoperability solutions. The company markets HIEBus™, a health care interoperability platform to enable edge applications to share clinical information in a secure, reliable, and incremental manner. Offering core capabilities like a community-wide master patient index, terminology standardization, episode grouping, and advanced analytics, HIEBus powers statewide and regional exchanges, regional care coordination networks, provider-centric clinical integration initiatives, and multicenter observational data studies. Dr. Kheterpal is very active in the interoperability and health information technology landscape and serves as technical director of the South Carolina Health Information Exchange. Previously, Dr. Kheterpal served as the global general manager and vice president for clinical information systems for GE Healthcare, where he led GE's clinical IT initiatives. Dr. Kheterpal received his doctorate in medicine from the University of Michigan at Ann Arbor, where he also earned a bachelor's degree in biomedical sciences.

Rebecca Daniels Kush, PhD, is a founder and the current president and CEO of the Clinical Data Interchange Standards Consortium. Dr. Kush has more than 25 years of experience in the area of clinical research. She has worked for the National Institutes of Health, academia, a global contract research organization, and pharmaceutical companies in the United States and Japan. Among numerous publications, Dr. Kush is lead author of the book *eClinical Trials: Planning and Implementation.* Dr. Kush has given invited presentations (including keynotes) and tutorials at industry conferences, the Food and Drug Administration, and other venues in the United States, Europe, and Japan for more than 20 years. She earned a PhD in physiology and pharmacology from the University of California, San Diego, School of Medicine in La Jolla, California, and has a BS in chemistry and biology from the University of New Mexico.

Marty LaVenture, PhD, MDH, is director of the Office of Health Information Technology and e-Health at the Minnesota Department of Health. Dr. LaVenture is currently leading the statewide Minnesota e-Health Initiative and directs the department's Center for Health Informatics. Current projects include models for e-health profiles, assessment of EHR adoption, and work as lead author for the revised chapter on public health informatics in upcoming fourth edition of Shortliffe and Cimino's *Textbook of Biomedical Informatics.* Dr. LaVenture has a master's degree in epidemiology and a PhD in health informatics from the University of Minnesota. Previously, he served as the assistant state epidemiologist for Wisconsin Division of Health, and he has also worked for a national private medical software corporation. Dr. LaVenture is currently an adjunct member of the health informatics faculty at the University of Minnesota. In 2008, he was named as one of the top 100 influential health leaders in Minnesota. Nationally, Dr. LaVenture serves on the editorial board for the *Journal of Biomedical Informatics.* He is a member of the Association of State and Territorial Health Officials ehealth policy committee. Dr. LaVenture has authored or co-authored many articles and scientific publications, delivered numerous presentations to state and national audiences, and received multiple awards for his work and accomplishments. He is an elected fellow of the American College of Medical Informatics.

Mark Leenay, MS, MD, is one of our nation's experts on geriatrics and hospice and palliative care and is the chief medical officer and senior vice president at OptumHealth Care Solutions. As chief medical officer, he oversees all clinical programs, ranging from wellness to the most complex medical conditions. He leads the clinical performance team, which is accountable for clinical care and quality in the company's wellness, case management, and disease management programs, as well as the clinical performance of external provider partners. Dr. Leenay's focus is providing members the best care from experienced and knowledgeable providers, leading to shorter hospital stays and improved health. He achieves these goals by championing exceptional performance within OptumHealth's Centers of Excellence and other clinical networks. Previously, Dr. Leenay was chief medical officer for the Medicare and retirement business for United Healthcare, with accountability for clinical programs, medical payment policy, and network relationships. Prior to joining UnitedHealth Group in 2006, Mark directed the palliative care division at the University of Minnesota, Fairview. Mark received his MD from Thomas Jefferson University and completed his residency at Overlook Hospital, an affiliate of Columbia University. He earned his bachelor's degree from LeMoyne College and his master's degree in psychology from the University of Pennsylvania. Mark is board-certified in family medicine, geriatrics, and hospice and palliative care. He is a board member of the Long Term Quality Alliance and sits on the quality and research committees of the National Hospice and Palliative Care Association. He is a former director of the board of the American Academy of Hospice and Palliative Medicine.

Mia A. Levy, MD, PhD, is the director of cancer clinical informatics for the Vanderbilt-Ingram Cancer Center and an assistant professor of biomedical informatics and medicine. Dr. Levy received her undergraduate degree in bioengineering from the University of Pennsylvania in 1997 and her medical doctorate from Rush University in 2003. She then spent 6 years at Stanford University completing postgraduate training in internal medicine and medical oncology while completing her PhD in biomedical informatics. She joined the faculty at Vanderbilt as an assistant professor in biomedical informatics and medicine in August 2009. She is a practicing medical oncologist specializing in the treatment of breast cancer. Dr. Levy's research interests include biomedical informatics methods to support the continuum of cancer care and cancer research. Her current research projects include informatics methods for (1) image-based cancer treatment response assessment using quantitative imaging, (2) clinical decision support for treatment prioritization of molecular subtypes of cancer, (3) protocol-based plan management, and (4) learning cancer systems.

David Madigan, PhD, is professor and chair of statistics at Columbia University in New York City. He received a bachelor's degree in mathematical sciences and a PhD in statistics, both from Trinity College, Dublin. He has previously worked for AT&T Inc., Soliloquy Inc., the University of Washington, Rutgers University, and SkillSoft, Inc. He has more than 100 publications in areas such as Bayesian statistics, text mining, Monte Carlo methods, pharmacovigilance, and probabilistic graphical models. He is an elected fellow of the American Statistical Association and of the Institute of Mathematical Statistics. He has just finished a term as editor-in-chief of *Statistical Science*.

Carol J. McCall, FSA, MAAA, is the chief strategy officer for GNS Healthcare, a big-data analytics company whose industrialized knowledge discovery platform extracts cause-effect relationships directly and at scale from observational data. Her personal goal is to leverage these capabilities to redesign the entire notion of "evidence" and ignite a true learning system in the health care system. Prior to joining GNS Healthcare, Ms. McCall was chief innovation officer for Tenzing Health, a subsidiary of Vanguard Health Systems, where she merged creative analytic approaches with human-centered design. Building team-based care models whose approach extended into the community, these approaches were shown to materially improve health, dramatically reduce costs, and open new opportunities in a community's economic sustainability. At Humana, Ms. McCall led R&D efforts in the Innovation Center, where she pioneered sophisticated analytics to build a diverse portfolio of prediction, knowledge discovery, and simulation models. She also launched Humana's innovations in personalized medicine, led Humana's Health Services Research Center (HSRC), and helped launch Green Ribbon Health, LLC, a Florida-based company with innovations in health support services for seniors, later serving on its board of directors. In other roles at Humana, Ms. McCall served as chief information officer and as vice president, pharmacy management. Outside of Humana, she served as executive vice president of managed care business development for Allscripts Healthcare Solutions and as an actuarial consultant for Milliman, where she helped fashion novel risk-sharing arrangements and implement risk-adjustment methodologies. In policy and advisory roles, Ms. McCall served a 4-year term as member of the nation's National Committee on Vital and Health Statistics, served as an advisor to the HRP Scientific Program Board, and was a member of the HSRC's governing board. She currently sits on the advisory board of Keas, a consumer health company. Ms. McCall is a fellow of the Society of Actuaries and a member of the American Academy of Actuaries.

Farzad Mostashari, MD, ScM, serves as national coordinator for health information technology within the Office of the National Coordinator for Health Information Technology (ONC) at the Department of Health and Human Services. Dr. Farzad joined ONC in July 2009. Previously, he served at the New York City Department of Health and Mental Hygiene as assistant commissioner for the Primary Care Information Project, where he facilitated the adoption of prevention-oriented health information technology by more than 1,500 providers in underserved communities. Dr. Mostashari also led the Centers for Disease Control and Prevention (CDC)-funded NYC Center of Excellence in Public Health Informatics and an Agency for Healthcare Research and Quality–funded project focused on quality measurement at the point of care. Prior to this, he established the Bureau of Epidemiology Services at the NYC Department of Health, charged with providing epidemiologic and statistical expertise and data for decision making to the health department. Dr. Mostashari completed his graduate training at the Harvard School of Public Health and Yale Medical School and his internal medicine residency at Massachusetts General Hospital, and completed the CDC's Epidemic Intelligence Service. He was one of the lead investigators in the outbreaks of West Nile Virus and anthrax in New York City, and among the first developers of real-time electronic disease surveillance systems nationwide.

J. Marc Overhage, MD, PhD, is the chief medical informatics officer for Siemens Healthcare. Prior to joining Siemens, he was the founding chief executive officer of the Indiana Health Information Exchange, director of medical informatics at the Regenstrief Institute, Inc., and a Sam Regenstrief Professor of Medical Informatics at the Indiana University School of Medicine. He has spent more than 25 years developing and implementing scientific and clinical systems and evaluating their value. With his colleagues from the Regenstrief Institute, he created a community-wide electronic medical record (called the Indiana Network for Patient Care) containing data from many sources, including laboratories, pharmacies, and hospitals in central Indiana. The system currently connects a majority of acute care hospitals in Indiana and includes inpatient and outpatient encounter data, laboratory results, immunization data, and other selected data for 12 million patients. In order to create a sustainable financial model, he helped create the Indiana Health Information Exchange, a not-for-profit corporation. In addition, Dr. Overhage has developed and evaluated clinical decision support, including inpatient and outpatient computerized physician order entry and the underlying knowledge bases to support them. He practiced general internal medicine for more than 20 years, including the ambulatory, inpatient, and emergency care settings. During the past decade, Dr. Overhage has played a significant regional and national leadership role in advancing the policy, standards, financing, and implementation of health information exchange. He serves on the Health Information Technology Standards Committee as well as the board of directors of the National Quality Forum, and is engaged in a number of national health care initiatives.

Richard Platt, MD, MSc, is professor and chair of the department of population medicine at Harvard Medical School and the Harvard Pilgrim Health Care Institute. He is principal investigator of the Food and Drug Administration's (FDA's) Mini-Sentinel program, of contracts with FDA's Center for Drugs Evaluation and Research and Center for Biologics Evaluation and Research to conduct postmarketing studies of drugs and biologics' safety and effectiveness. He chaired the FDA's Drug Safety and Risk Management Advisory Committee and is a member of the Association of American Medical Colleges' Advisory Panel on Research and the Institute of Medicine's Roundtable on Value & Science-Driven Health Care. Dr. Platt was co-chair of the board of scientific counselors of the Centers for Disease Control and Prevention's (CDC's) Center for Infectious Diseases. Additionally, he has chaired the National Institutes of Health epidemiology study section and Disease Control 2, and the CDC Office of Health Care Partnerships steering committee. Dr. Platt is also principal investigator of a CDC Center of Excellence in Public Health Informatics, the Agency for Healthcare Research and Quality (AHRQ) HMO Research Network Center for Education and Research in Therapeutics, the AHRQ HMO Research Network DEcIDE Center, and the CDC Eastern Massachusetts Prevention Epicenter.

Appendix B

Workshop Agenda

DIGITAL DATA PRIORITIES FOR CONTINUOUS LEARNING IN HEALTH AND HEALTH CARE

An Institute of Medicine Workshop
Sponsored by the Office of the National Coordinator for Health Information Technology

MARCH 23, 2012

KECK CENTER
500 FIFTH STREET NW, WASHINGTON DC 20001

A LEARNING HEALTH SYSTEM ACTIVITY
IOM ROUNDTABLE ON VALUE & SCIENCE-DRIVEN HEALTH CARE

Meeting objectives

1. Discuss the current quality status of digital health data.
2. Explore challenges, and identify key questions related to data quality in the use of EHRs, patient registries, administrative data, and public health sources for learning—continuous and episodic—and for system operational and improvement purposes.
3. Engage individuals and organizations leading the way in improving the reliability, availability, and usability of digital health data for real-time knowledge generation and health improvement in a continuously learning health system.
4. Identify and characterize the current deficiencies and consider strategies, priorities, and responsibilities to address the deficiencies.
5. Initiate the development of a strategic framework for integrated and networked stewardship of efforts to continuously increase digital data utility.

Agenda

7:30 am   Coffee and light breakfast available

8:00 am   **Welcome, introductions, and overview**
Welcome, framing of the meeting and agenda overview
- J. Michael McGinnis (Institute of Medicine)
- Farzad Mostashari (Office of the National Coordinator)
- James Walker (Planning Committee Chair)

8:15 am   **Characteristics, challenges, and determinants of data quality**

> ➤ **Session Description:** This session includes brief comments on the data quality challenges that lie ahead and a longer discussion of the characteristics and determinants of digital health data quality.

> ➤ **Key Topics:**
> - Challenges on the horizon
>   *Doug Fridsma (ONC)*
> - Characteristics and determinants of data quality
>   *Marc Overhage (Siemens)*

OPEN DISCUSSION

9:00 am   **Performance assessment**

> ➤ **Session Description:** This session focuses on the quality of digital health data needed to evaluate clinical care delivery, population management and the business and operating processes that make up a learning health system.

> ➤ **Key Topics:**
> - Assessing value
>   *Carol McCall (GNS)*
> - Managing populations and processes
>   *Mark Leenay (OptumHealth)*

OPEN DISCUSSION

10:00 am   Break

APPENDIX B   59

10:15 am   **Enabling research**

   ➤ **Session Description:** This session focuses on the quality of digital health data needed to enable research.

   ➤ **Key Topics:**
   - Clinical research
     Rebecca Kush (Clinical Data Interchange Standards Consortium)
   - Translational informatics
     Mia Levy (Vanderbilt)

   OPEN DISCUSSION

11:15 am   **Supporting public health and surveillance**

   ➤ **Session Description:** This session focuses on the quality of digital health data needed to support of public health functions, including surveillance.

   ➤ **Key Topics:**
   - Public health surveillance and management
     James Buehler (CDC)
   - State-level perspective
     Martin LaVenture (Minnesota Department of Health)

   OPEN DISCUSSION

12:15 pm   **Lunch keynote**

   Who is your customer?
   James Heywood, PatientsLikeMe

1:00 pm   **Approaches to continuous improvement using large-scale datasets**

   ➤ **Session Description:** Session presentations will focus on the implications of digital health data quality on the potential for learning from large amounts of health data.

> Key Topics:
>   o Using distributed data/Query Health
>   *Rich Platt (Harvard) and Rich Elmore (ONC)*
>   o Data analysis and discovery of significant patterns
>   *David Madigan (OMOP/Columbia)*

OPEN DISCUSSION

2:00 pm **Innovative approaches to addressing data challenges**

> **Session Description:** This session will focus on innovative approaches to overcoming some prominent challenges associated with using health data.

> Topics:
>   o Data harmonization
>   *Chris Chute (Mayo)*
>   o Linking data across time and sources
>   *Vik Kheterpal (CareEvolution Inc.)*

OPEN DISCUSSION

3:00 pm **Strategies going forward**

> **Session Description:** This session will include a rapid-fire, moderated discussion to identify the top 10 actions necessary for progress discussed during the course of the meeting.

> 1. Identification of potential action steps—20 min. (45 seconds each)
> 2. Rapid identification of pros and cons—15 min.
> 3. Identification of top ten leading action steps—25 min.

OPEN DISCUSSION

4:00 pm **Next steps**

> **Session Description:** This session will build off of the 10 action steps identified in the previous session and outline options to move forward.

5:00 pm **Adjourn**